Preventing and Reversing Heart Disease

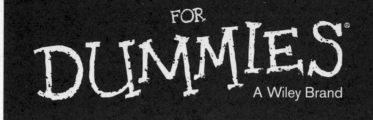
FOR
DUMMIES®
A Wiley Brand

by James M. Rippe, MD

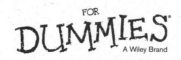
FOR
DUMMIES®
A Wiley Brand

Preventing and Reversing Heart Disease For Dummies®

Published by: **John Wiley & Sons, Inc.,** 111 River Street, Hoboken, NJ 07030-5774, www.wiley.com

Copyright © 2015 by John Wiley & Sons, Inc., Hoboken, New Jersey

Published simultaneously in Canada

For general information on our other products and services, please contact our Customer Care Department within the U.S. at 877-762-2974, outside the U.S. at 317-572-3993, or fax 317-572-4002. For technical support, please visit www.wiley.com/techsupport.

Wiley publishes in a variety of print and electronic formats and by print-on-demand. Some material included with standard print versions of this book may not be included in e-books or in print-on-demand. If this book refers to media such as a CD or DVD that is not included in the version you purchased, you may download this material at http://booksupport.wiley.com. For more information about Wiley products, visit www.wiley.com.

Library of Congress Control Number: 2014948558

ISBN 978-1-118-94423-3 (pbk); ISBN 978-1-118-94424-0 (ebk); ISBN 978-1-118-94425-7

Manufactured in the United States of America

10 9 8 7 6 5 4 3 2 1

Contents at a Glance

Recipes at a Glance

Soups, Salads, and Sauces

Breakfast Items

Smoothies, Shakes, and Tea

Table of Contents

Introduction

· ·

As you read this book, your heart is beating away in your chest, sustaining your life. Although it's about the size of a clenched adult fist and weighs less than a pound, your heart beats 40 million times a year and generates enough force to lift you 100 miles into the atmosphere. What an amazing — and absolutely essential — machine!

So consider these facts:

- ✔ One American dies of heart disease every 40 seconds — amounting to almost 600,000 deaths every year.
- ✔ Almost every American adult has at least one of these risk factors for heart disease: high blood pressure, high total cholesterol or LDL cholesterol, smoking, being overweight, diabetes, stress, physical inactivity, or nutrient-poor diet. Not one family in America is left untouched by heart disease.

But here's the good news: Regardless of your age, sex, ethnicity, and current heart health, you can acquire the knowledge and take action to work toward a healthier heart and the benefits that go with it. This book will help.

About This Book

Preventing and Reversing Heart Disease For Dummies is a commonsense guide for everyone. It discusses simple things that you can do every day to maximize your cardiac health and prevent heart disease. You'll also find some basic strategies and lifestyle practices to reduce and reverse the risk factors you may have for the major forms of heart disease.

If you (or a loved one) already have heart disease, you also have come to the right place. I explore some facts related to coronary heart disease, angina, heart attacks, hypertension, heart failure, and many other cardiac conditions. You'll discover ways to work with your doctor to control these conditions and possibly to reverse many of their consequences. Lifestyle modifications provide the foundation for effective change.

There are a few things that you should know about how I put the book together. First, you can read the first part of the book (Chapters 1 to 3) for a brief but comprehensive introduction to heart disease and then go to the chapters that interest you most. Or you can go right to a specific chapter that you need, such as Chapter 5 on creating a beneficial nutrition and physical activity plan or Chapter 9 on managing cholesterol problems. Part V contains more than 40 dishes you can choose from to start making more heart-healthy meals right away. If you want to skip sidebars (where I provide additional tips) or Technical Stuff icons, that's okay, too. Think of this book as a tool that you can use any way that works best for you.

You will find it helpful to note a few conventions I use:

- *Atherosclerosis* is the medical name for the cardiovascular disease process that starts with fatty streaks in the arteries and progresses to large lesions that narrow the arteries and may rupture and form clots that block arteries.

- When atherosclerosis occurs in the arteries of the heart, it is called *coronary heart disease* and abbreviated *CHD*. This is the common term I use throughout the book, although this condition is also called *coronary artery disease (CAD)*.

- In the recipe section, temperatures are Fahrenheit, *olive oil* is extra virgin olive oil, and pepper is ideally freshly ground (but that's optional). (See the appendix for a metric conversion chart.)

- ☺ This icon highlights vegetarian recipes.

Within this book, some web addresses may break across two lines of text. If you are reading a print copy of this book and want to go to the website, simply key in the web address exactly as it's printed in the text, ignoring the line break. If you are reading this as an e-book, just click on the link to go directly to the web page.

Foolish Assumptions

Every writer envisions the people who will read his (or her) book. Here are some qualities that I think you have:

- You care about your heart health and that of your family. And you want up-to-date and practical information that will help you take steps to ensure heart health.

- You are not afraid to take action to improve your health. And you want practical steps.

- You wish to increase your knowledge about heart disease and how to decrease your risk of specific conditions that lead to heart disease.

- You want to work as a partner with your doctor(s).

✔ You realize that a healthy lifestyle, not medicines or medical procedures, is the foundation of overall health, including heart health.

✔ You are ready to commit to creating new healthful habits and taking control of your heart health.

Icons Used in This Book

This book uses the following icons to point out different kinds of information:

This icon provides detailed information about how the heart works, what is going on in the body and heart when a cardiac event happens, or how a procedure works or what it does. But don't worry — all technical stuff is presented in plain English.

This icon signals key information about the conditions that are risk factors for heart disease and about specific heart diseases. It also highlights key information about heart health that is worth remembering long after you put this book down.

This icon indicates practical suggestions you can put to work to help you reach your heart-health goals.

Think of this icon as a caution flag. It points out things or practices that may be harmful to heart health or overall health.

Beyond the Book

"But wait there's more . . . !" Don't you hate those infomercials? I'm happy to say that the extras that come with this book actually give you brief "stuff" you can use.

Need the basic steps and tips for keeping your heart healthy? Need to refresh your memory of nutrient-rich foods before you hit the deli? Need a little inspiration to work some exercise into your day? Got a check up and need to know what to ask the doctor? Access the Cheat Sheet at www.dummies.com/cheatsheet/preventingreversingheartdisease.

Each part of the book also has additional online articles. You can find tools for managing weight, tips for eating out, a checklist of essential equipment for your kitchen, and more. Head to www.dummies.com/extras/preventing reversingheartdisease.

Where to Go from Here

As I note earlier, you can start with any chapter you like in this book. The simplest approach — and one that refreshes your understanding of the basics of heart health and the risks of heart disease — is to start by reading (or skimming through) Part I and then go to the chapters that most interest you or answer your current questions.

If your primary interest is adopting a heart-healthy way of eating and increasing your physical activity, then start with Chapter 5 which tells you how to embrace a healthy diet and lifestyle. If you also want to lose weight, then head on over to Chapter 10 on managing weight. Or if you have received a diagnosis of high blood pressure (Chapter 8) or of high cholesterol problems (Chapter 9), you can get immediate information and tips in those chapters.

Couples starting a family or raising one want the best health for their children. Overall health and heart health are family affairs. Chapters 7 and 23 give you invaluable tips.

Just as there are many habits and conditions that put your heart as risk, there are many pathways to heart health. This book opens the gate to these pathways. So here's my invitation to take the first step on the path that works for you.

Part I
Getting Started with Preventing and Reversing Heart Disease

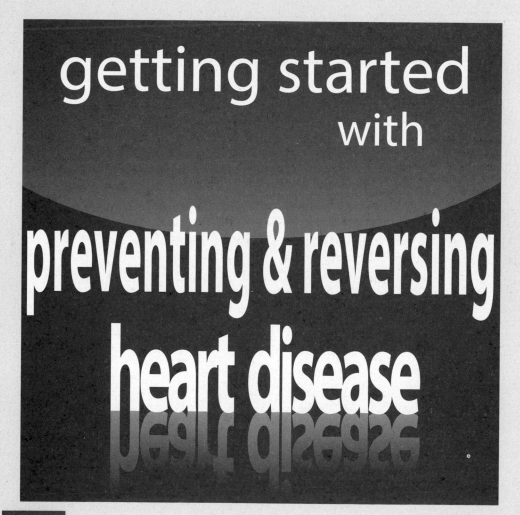

In this part . . .

- ✔ Find the basic information you need to begin taking control of your heart health.

- ✔ Understand how heart disease can affect your life and what you can do about it.

- ✔ Discover how the miracle machine that is your heart works and how heart disease develops.

- ✔ Look at how heart disease progresses to such events as chest pain or heart attacks.

- ✔ Find out what behaviors and conditions increase your risk of developing heart disease and what you can do to stop these risks in their tracks.

Chapter 1

Taking Charge of Your Heart Health

. . . .

. . . .

*H*uman health, daily performance, and life itself depend on the heart. The heart and the cardiovascular system have amazing sophistication, strength, and durability. At the same time, the health of the heart rests in a fragile balance. When even small parts of its complex machinery are a little bit out of whack, the heart can cause great discomfort, pain, and even death.

Despite the emotional energy we attach to our hearts and the heart's crucial importance to life itself, most people are pretty ignorant about the heart and how it works. You know you can't live without one. You know that heart disease is pretty common and more than a little scary. So when your doctor says your cholesterol levels or elevated blood pressure are raising your risk of heart disease, it's a little alarming. And the bottom falls out of your stomach if your physician says, "I don't think that chest pain is a muscle strain. We'd better do some tests to rule out heart disease." At moments like that, you wish you knew more about that small pump thumping away in your chest and all the things that threaten it and what you can do about them. That's where *Preventing and Reversing Heart Disease For Dummies* comes in.

In this chapter, I show you first why heart disease is such an important health problem for Americans and why you should care about that. More important, however, I give you an overview of how possible it is to prevent heart disease for you and your family. Even if you already have risk factors for heart disease or have been diagnosed with heart disease, you will see that you can take steps to reverse these risks and to control or even reduce some symptoms or manifestations of heart disease. This chapter outlines the good news and practical strategies that I discuss in detail in each chapter in this book.

Facing the Bad News about Heart Disease

Heart disease is public health enemy number one in America. In one or another of its manifestations, heart disease touches virtually every family in the United States. Although the death rate from heart disease in the U.S. has been declining steadily — about 31 percent between 2000 and 2010 — the health burden and danger of heart disease remains alarmingly high. Consider these startling facts:

- Almost 84 million Americans — more than one in every four — have one or more types of heart disease.

- Heart disease and stroke cause more than one of every three deaths.

- Heart disease is an equal-opportunity killer. It is the leading cause of death in men and women and all ethnic and racial groups in the United States.

- About 150,000 deaths from heart disease occur annually in people younger than 65. Preventable deaths in this younger population have not declined significantly in the last 10 years.

- While deaths from heart disease declined, the numbers of operations and procedures for heart disease increased 28 percent between 2000 and 2010.

- If money is the most important thing in your life, you might like to know that the yearly estimated cost of cardiovascular disease in the United States is $315.4 *billion.*

As a cardiologist, I've seen these statistics made all too real in the lives of too many patients. But I've also seen what people can do to take charge of heart health at all stages, from working to lower their risk of developing heart disease to learning how to control and live well with advanced coronary heart disease (CHD) and its varied manifestations.

Seizing the Good News about Preventing Heart Disease

The bad-news facts about heart disease are real, but they aren't the only news. Extensive research proves that you can do many things in your daily life and in working with your physician to use the latest medical science in order to preserve and maximize the health of your heart — even if you already have heart disease. Consider these good-news facts:

✔ People who are physically active on a regular basis cut their risk of heart disease in half.

✔ People who stop smoking cigarettes can return their risk of heart disease and stroke to almost normal levels within five years after stopping.

✔ Overweight people who lose as little as 5 to 10 percent of their body weight can substantially lower their risk of heart disease. In Chapter 10, I offer suggestions that can help you maintain or reclaim a healthy body weight, and in Part V, I offer a number of recipes that prove you don't have to deny yourself enjoyable foods to do so.

✔ Simple changes in what you eat can lower total blood cholesterol and LDL-cholesterol, both of which contribute to heart disease.

✔ The number of deaths from heart disease declined by millions during the last decade — a decline largely based on lifestyle changes.

Checking Out Heart Disease as an Equal Opportunity Health Problem

So who should care about heart disease? As the previous sections suggest, everyone. No matter your present state of heart health, you can do plenty to reduce your risk factors for heart disease. (Find out more about that in Chapter 3.) You need to care about heart disease whether you are young or old, man or woman, totally healthy or coping with heart disease or other health problems, and regardless of your ethnic and racial background. If you belong to certain groups, however, some associated facts and conditions should raise your consciousness about why paying attention to heart disease and heart health should be important to you.

If you're an adult younger than 65

If you think of heart disease as a problem mainly for older adults, that's understandable. The majority of deaths from heart disease do occur in people older than 65. However, as I discuss in Chapter 2, early signs of fatty streaks and fibrous plaques, the precursors of coronary artery disease, are already present in a majority of young adults between the ages of 21 and 39. Here are some other reasons that younger adults should take steps now to prevent heart disease:

✔ About half of all sudden cardiac arrests occur in people under age 65, many in people in their 40s and 50s.

✔ 34 percent of people hospitalized for stroke are younger than age 65.

✔ More than 1 in 5 Americans with heart failure are younger than age 60.

✔ An estimated 80 percent of premature heart disease and stroke is preventable.

✔ Among U.S. youth and adults aged 12 to 60, almost none meet the seven criteria for ideal heart health established by the American Heart Association. That figure would be none, except that 0.3 percent of young adults ages 20 to 29 meet the seven ideal criteria.

So if you are younger than 65, there is no time like the present to start taking steps toward better heart health.

If you're a woman

Although heart disease is an equal-opportunity killer, many people, men and women alike, continue to think that heart disease is primarily a *man's* problem. Wrong! Consider these facts:

✔ Although men suffer heart attacks an average of ten years earlier than women, after menopause, women catch up. Within the year after a heart attack, 42 percent of women will die, compared to 24 percent of men.

✔ In spite of extensive public education campaigns, only 54 percent of women know that heart disease is the leading cause of death for women. Heart disease kills more women than all forms of cancer combined.

✔ Stress poses a greater risk of heart disease in women than in men.

✔ Diabetes in women is a greater risk factor for heart disease than it is in men.

In the final analysis, heart disease is at least as dangerous for women as it is for men. So, if you're a woman who bought this book for the man in your life, think again. Keep this copy for yourself and buy another one for him! There is just as much in this book for you as there is for the men in your life.

If you're African American

Heart disease is the leading cause of death for African Americans, just as it is for all Americans. Although every individual is different, African Americans, as a group, experience a higher incidence of certain conditions that contribute to the risk of heart disease. Consider these facts:

✔ African Americans develop high blood pressure at earlier ages than white Americans, and at any decade of life, more have high blood pressure, which is a risk factor for heart disease and stroke. Currently, among African Americans, 47 percent of women and 43 percent of men have high blood pressure, compared to 31 percent of women and 33 percent of men among white Americans.

✔ Compared to white Americans, African Americans have twice the risk of a first stroke and are more likely to die from the stroke.

✔ African Americans are 1.7 times as likely as non-Hispanic whites to have diabetes, a factor that contributes to developing heart disease. They are also more likely to have complications, such as blindness or kidney failure.

Although much current research seeks to determine the causes of the higher incidence of risk factors, such as high blood pressure, among African Americans, African Americans can prevent and control hypertension and other risk factors by adopting appropriate lifestyle practices and working with their physicians to develop appropriate drug therapies.

If you're a parent

The incidence of heart disease is, of course, very rare among children and youths. But the roots of heart disease are firmly planted in childhood. As people in the United States have spent more and more time in front of the TV or computer screen, commuting in cars, and eating out, children in the U.S. are learning lifestyle behaviors and developing health conditions that may make them more, rather than less, likely to develop heart disease and other health problems. The good (and bad) habits of a lifetime usually begin in childhood. Parents need to set good examples for their children and encourage them to adopt practices that optimize their future health. Consider the following facts about children in the U.S.:

✔ An estimated 2.4 million teenagers ages 12 to 17 use tobacco products. Though this figure has declined significantly in the last decade, 23.4 percent of high school students currently use tobacco products. Smoking is a major contributor to heart disease, cancer, and other health problems.

✔ Approximately 50 percent of American teenagers get no regular physical activity.

✔ Approximately 17 percent of children and youths, ages 2 to 19, are obese, another risk factor for heart disease.

To find out how you can teach your children heart-healthy habits that will last a lifetime, head to Chapter 7.

If you're older

Unfortunately, many Americans expect heart trouble to be part of their older years. That need not be so. And if you *are* older and, for that matter, even if you already have heart disease, you can do plenty to avoid being part of these statistics:

- Approximately 80 percent of deaths from heart disease occur in people older than 65.

- More than 70 percent of men and women aged 60 to 79 have cardiovascular disease. For people age 80 and older, the percentage having heart disease rises to 83 percent of men and 87 percent of women.

- After age 55, the incidence of stroke doubles with each decade of life.

- Two of the most frequent causes of hospitalization for older adults are coronary atherosclerosis and congestive heart failure.

Reversing the Risks for Heart Disease

No matter what your overall health now — even if you already have heart disease or have had a heart attack — clinical research shows that working to reduce your risk factors for heart disease can greatly reduce your risks of developing heart disease, help you to halt the progression of atherosclerosis, and, if you have had a heart event, greatly reduce the risk of a second event. Take a look at what research reveals about how you can improve your health:

- If you have a diagnosis of atherosclerosis or symptoms of coronary heart disease, modifying risk factors such as high blood pressure, blood cholesterol problems, physical inactivity, and being overweight can reduce your risk of a future heart attack or the need for coronary artery angioplasty or bypass surgery, and add years to your life. With lifestyle modifications and appropriate medical therapies, many individuals can bring all these risks back into the healthy range.

- Appropriate physical activity or exercise improves the ability to perform activities comfortably for people with angina and people who've had heart attacks or even coronary surgery.

- Weight loss can help control cholesterol levels, blood pressure, and diabetes — conditions that contribute to the continued progress of heart disease.

- If you smoke and have had a heart attack, quitting smoking significantly reduces your risk of having a second heart attack or experiencing sudden death.

✔ Over the last 30 years, a number of studies examining the possibility of reversing atherosclerosis, the narrowing of the coronary arteries, suggest that rigorous lifestyle modifications supported by appropriate medications can halt the progression of atherosclerosis and may lead to a degree of regression of atherosclerosis for many individuals.

You can find strategies for tackling several of these risk factors in Part II.

Reversing Heart Disease — Hope or Hype?

When Thomas Wolfe's famous novel *You Can't Go Home Again* came out in 1940, most people thought his title had hit on one true thing. For many years, cardiologists believed that same truth applied to coronary heart disease: Once you had this progressive, relentless condition, you might be able to slow down the process, but you couldn't actually reverse it — you couldn't go home again.

But in medicine, as in life, the quest to go home again continues. Cardiologists now know that *yes*, you can control a number of contributing risk factors to heart disease and thus, for many people, halt the progression of CHD in its tracks. If you have coronary heart disease and want to make this happen, however, you're going to have to stop cold and make major changes in how you eat, exercise, work, and generally live your life. You usually have to take lipid-lowering (cholesterol and other fats) medicines, too. But as long as you're willing to do your part and adopt these strict measures, you can look forward to more hope than hype in the promise that you can stop your CHD where it is. In some cases, you may even be able to reduce the lesions, called plaque, that grow in the artery walls and that result in narrowed arteries and ruptures and clots that cause heart disease and heart attacks.

Before going any further, I want to emphasize two points. If you're thinking that, given the good news, you can live a life of sin (sloth and gluttony of the seven deadly sins come to mind) and then later repent and turn the negative health effects around, forget about it! Preventing heart disease is always better than to trying to stop it or reverse it. Likewise, this book is not a do-it-yourself manual if you have symptoms of heart disease or have been diagnosed with it. You need to work with your cardiologist.

Can coronary artery disease regress? There isn't a simple answer to this question. But a number of studies in animals and humans show promise. The goal of reversing heart disease doesn't just require reducing the amount and size of the narrowings in coronary arteries; it also requires that the lining of the arteries, called the *endothelium,* be restored to its normal function, that inflammation be controlled, and that many of the physiological entities that contribute to the progression of heart disease be returned to their proper function. You can see how complicated this process is going to be. (You can read more about how coronary heart disease develops in Chapter 2.)

The lifestyle strategies this book details will typically help you prevent heart disease and manage and even reverse any risk factors for heart disease that you have. However, many people will require not only significant lifestyle modifications but also the appropriate medications to lower their risks. That's why you should always work with your doctor to have regular checkups. Then, if you are diagnosed with risks for heart disease or with heart disease itself, you and your doctor can work as partners to plan the best therapeutic program for you. Research is bringing new insights all the time, and your cardiologist will be your best source of up-to-date strategies. Head to Part IV for information about medications, surgical options, and complementary therapies used for heart disease.

Taking Charge of Your Heart Health

Without question, heart disease is a serious enemy. In fact, it's the biggest enemy. But you can take charge of your heart health, whatever its present state.

As I often like to say: *Ipsa scientia potestas est,* or knowledge is power. For that reason, the remainder of this book is full of information that can empower you to understand the basics about heart health and heart disease and partner with your physician in putting the power of simple lifestyle practices and medical technology to work for you. Taking control of your heart health offers other wonderful upsides for living well that include the following:

- **Improving your overall health:** Many of the steps that benefit your heart health also improve your total health and fitness, to say nothing of your good looks.

- **Increasing functionality:** Use it or lose it, goes the old saying. The healthier your heart, the greater the probability that you can stay active, mobile, and engaged in pursuits that interest you for a long, long time.

- **Increasing economic benefits:** The healthier you are, the lower your healthcare costs, and the more money in your pocket for fun things.

- **Increasing longevity:** Keeping your heart healthy is not an iron-clad guarantee that you'll live longer, but considering the mortality rates of people with heart disease (reviewed earlier in this chapter), even card-carrying "Dummies" can figure out that keeping your heart as healthy as possible can keep the Grim Reaper away longer.

- **Having more fun:** Nothing slows you down or scares the family like a heart attack. Angina pain, angioplasty, coronary artery bypass surgery, and other common outcomes of heart disease aren't picnics in the park, either. Working for heart health and controlling heart disease can help you avoid these problems.

Chapter 2

Understanding the Onset and Outcomes of Heart Disease

In This Chapter

▶ Understanding what causes atherosclerosis and coronary heart disease

▶ Determining the causes and effects of angina

▶ Exploring what causes heart attacks

▶ Learning about arrhythmias, heart failure, and other forms of heart disease

*Y*our heart works harder than any other muscle in your body. Your life depends on this small but mighty pump never stopping. It's about the size of your clenched fist and weighs less than a pound. Depending on your age and physical condition, a normal heart beats 60 to 90 times per minute when you are sitting and may get up to 150 to 200+ times per minute when you are maxing out aerobic physical activity. A healthy heart is equipped to sustain at this pace for 70 to 90 years and beyond. The key word here is *healthy*.

From the moment you are born (and even before), multiple factors related to your biology, behavior, and environment have an impact, for good or ill, on your heart and cardiovascular system. Heart disease is progressive: It starts stealthily in the coronary (and other) arteries and progresses silently for years before any detectable signs of disease emerge. Research over the last 25 years provided new insights into how heart disease begins, starting at the cellular and molecular levels. These new insights are helping to prevent heart disease in the first place and to halt or, in some aspects, even reverse its progress.

In this chapter, I first present a brief overview of the heart and cardiovascular system. Then, I discuss the silent precursors and early stages of heart disease. Next, I look at *angina* and *unstable angina,* two types of chest pain that are often the first signs of heart disease for many people. Finally, I discuss how disease progression may result in heart attacks, arrhythmia (heart rhythm problems), heart failure, and other acute problems.

Touring the Heart and Cardiovascular System

Understanding how your heart and cardiovascular system work provides a foundation for understanding heart disease and its many manifestations. Even if you begin snoozing at the mere idea of technical stuff, don't forget that knowledge is power. These basics can help you do a better job of keeping your heart healthy.

Pumping for life: The heart's anatomy and function

The heart is located in the center of the chest cavity, just to the left of the midline of the body. Figure 2-1 illustrates the exterior of a healthy heart and Figure 2-2 illustrates the interior. You need to understand the following important parts:

- **The heart muscle:** Called the *myocardium* (*myo* = muscle and *cardium* = heart; pronounced my-o-*car*-dee-um), this muscle contracts and relaxes to pump blood throughout the cardiovascular system.

- **The coronary arteries:** Three large coronary arteries and their many branches deliver a continuous supply of oxygenated blood to the heart. Narrowing of these arteries causes chest pain; blockage causes heart attack.

- **The pumping chambers:** The heart's job is to pump blood to the lungs to get oxygen and to pump the oxygenated blood to the rest of the body. To fulfill these tasks, the heart has a left and a right side (shown in Figure 2-2), each with one main pumping chamber called a *ventricle* located in the lower part of it. Sitting above the left and right ventricles are two small booster pumps called *atria* (or *atrium*, when you're talking about just one).

The right ventricle pumps deoxygenated blood from the body to the lungs to receive a new supply of oxygen and back to the heart, through the left atrium to the left ventricle. The left ventricle pumps oxygenated blood through the arterial system to the rest of the body where it feeds every single living cell. Various disease conditions can damage each of these structures.

✔ **The valves:** Four valves regulate the flow of blood in and out of the heart and from chamber to chamber. They act a bit like cardiac traffic cops by directing the way blood flows, how much of it flows, and when to stop it from flowing. Disease and injury can cause heart valves to leak, narrow, or otherwise malfunction, disrupting the heart's ability to pump blood efficiently.

✔ **The electrical system:** This electrical system is controlled by a group of specialized cells that spontaneously discharge, sending electrical currents down specialized nerves and tissues, causing the heart to contract. When any of these electrical structures becomes diseased or disordered, *arrhythmias* (ay-*rith*-mee-uhz), or heart rhythm disturbances, occur.

✔ **The pericardium:** The entire heart is positioned in a thin sac called the *pericardium* (*peri* = around and *cardium* = heart; pronounced per-ry-*car*-dee-um). Fluid within the sac lubricates the constantly moving surfaces. Inflammation of the pericardium from an infection or other cause causes *pericarditis*. Build-up of excess fluid inside the pericardium can cause problems with how the heart functions, a condition called *cardiac tamponade.*

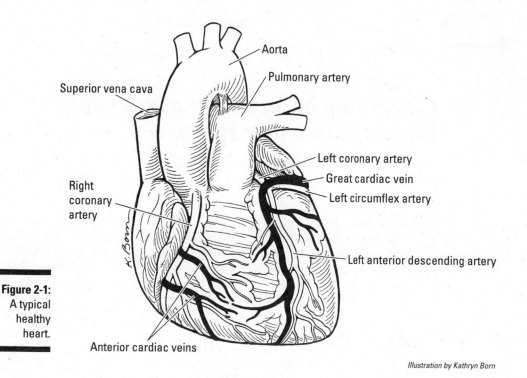

Figure 2-1:
A typical
healthy
heart.

Illustration by Kathryn Born

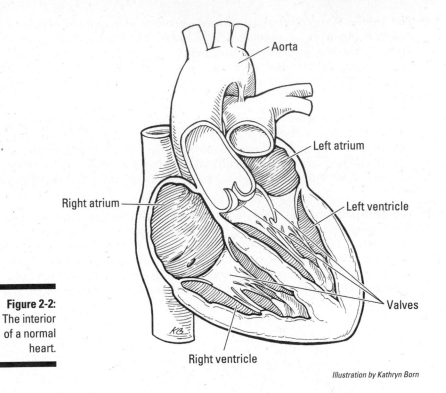

Aorta

Left atrium

Right atrium

Left ventricle

Valves

Figure 2-2:
The interior
of a normal
heart.

Right ventricle

Illustration by Kathryn Born

Connecting every cell in your body: The cardiovascular system

A pump is useless without the rest of the plumbing, which in your body is called the *cardiovascular system.* Here's a quick look at how it all fits together and functions.

✔ **The lungs:** The lungs are composed of an intricate series of air sacs surrounded by a complex, highly branching network of blood vessels. Their sole purpose is to receive the deoxygenated blood from the heart, fill the red corpuscles full of fresh oxygen, and send them back to the heart for delivery to the body. The red blood cells give off waste products such as carbon dioxide at the same time they take on oxygen; the lungs then expel the carbon dioxide. This low-pressure system facilitates the rapid flow and reoxygenation of enormous amounts of blood.

✔ **The arteries:** As oxygenated blood returns to the left side of the heart, it is pumped out to the body through the *aorta,* the main artery of the body, and into the rest of the arterial system to feed the entire body with oxygenated blood. Although the heart exerts enough force to push oxygenated blood throughout the body, the arteries also have muscular walls that help push the blood along. The force exerted against resistance of the artery walls creates a high-pressure system that is very *elastic* to allow the arteries to expand or contract to meet the needs of various organs and muscles. Your blood pressure reading results from measuring the pressure in these arteries when contracting and at rest. (Read more about high blood pressure in Chapter 8.)

✔ **The capillaries:** The arterial system divides and redivides into a system of ever smaller branches to distribute nourishing blood to each individual cell, ultimately ending up in a network of microscopic vessels called *capillaries,* which deliver oxygenated blood to the working cells of every organ and muscle in the body.

✔ **The veins:** After oxygen leaves the capillary system, the deoxygenated blood and waste products from the cells are carried back through the body in the *veins.* The veins ultimately come together in two very large veins, called the *inferior vena cava* (*vee*-nuh *cay*-vuh) and the *superior vena cava.* The inferior vena cava drains blood from the lower part of the body and superior vena cava drains blood from the upper part of the body. These veins discharge blood into the right atrium of the heart to be pumped into the right ventricle and out to the lungs again to start the whole process over again.

✔ **The blood:** Although blood is not considered part of the cardiovascular system, circulating blood to every cell of the body is the reason the cardiovascular system exists. This red fluid transports oxygen and fuel to the cells and removes waste products. It's also the delivery vehicle for many specialized cells and biochemicals, including those that contribute to the development of heart disease.

Keeping the beat: How the nervous system controls heart rate

In addition to its internal electrical system, the heart has profound linkages to the nervous system that provide additional control of the heart rate. Two main branches of the involuntary nervous system interact with the heart — the sympathetic nervous system and the parasympathetic nervous system. In simple terms, the *sympathetic nervous system* helps the heart speed up, and the *parasympathetic nervous system* helps the heart slow down. They act through direct nerve links to the heart and through the release of chemical substances that reach the heart through the bloodstream.

Understanding How Heart Disease Begins and Develops

The human cardiovascular system is wondrously complex. If every element is in balance and working as it should, a state called *homeostasis*, then the whole system, including the heart and blood vessels, would remain healthy. Unfortunately, multiple factors related to your biology and lifestyle can tip the system out of balance and trigger the development of heart disease. The earliest changes typically start in childhood or adolescence and then silently progress for years before producing changes that can be seen in diagnostic tests or symptoms that you experience. The most common type of cardiovascular disease is *atherosclerosis*.

Defining atherosclerosis — the most common form of cardiovascular disease

Atherosclerosis results from the gradual buildup of fatty deposits called *plaque,* or *lesions,* in the interior walls of large and medium-sized arteries. The disease process starts with small changes in the artery wall and takes years to develop to a point where the narrowing arteries may produce symptoms or negatively affect your health.

Narrowing in the heart's arteries leads to *coronary heart disease* (CHD), also called *coronary artery disease* (CAD). CHD gradually starves the heart muscle of the high level of oxygenated blood that it needs to function properly. A lack of adequate blood supply to the heart typically produces symptoms that range from angina and unstable angina (see "Recognizing angina, or chest pain" and "Defining Unstable Angina" later in this chapter) to heart attack or sudden death. Narrowing of the carotid arteries that carry blood to the brain increases your risk of stroke. Narrowed arteries in your legs or arms results in *peripheral artery disease* (PAD).

The term a*therosclerosis* comes from two Greek words — *athero* (paste, gruel) and *sclerosis* (hardness) — that may give you a graphic image of hardened sludge. Not a pretty picture, is it? But it's an apt image for these deposits of cholesterol, other fats, cellular wastes, platelets, calcium, and other substances. These deposits typically start with fatty streaks and grow to large bumps that distort the artery and block its interior where the blood must flow. Some plaques are stable and others are unstable or vulnerable to cracking or rupturing, which often leads to an artery-blocking blood clot and subsequent heart attack. The sections that follow profile that development process.

During the last 15 to 20 years, evidence from extensive population studies and clinical research has increased doctors' understanding of the many factors and pathways that contribute to the beginnings and progress of atherosclerosis. The next sections provide an overview of medical science's best understanding right now; however, you need to remember that new studies continually add to the knowledge of this complex, multifaceted disease.

Triggering the precursors of atherosclerosis

Biological factors that contribute to the development of cardiovascular disease are present from birth and perform vital functions that enable the human body to grow and resist infection. As a consequence, all human beings are born with the potential to develop heart disease. The early precursors of atherosclerosis frequently occur in children, teens, and young adults. Fortunately, adopting a heart-healthy lifestyle can usually reverse these early manifestations. The sooner you start, the better, but it's never too late.

Current biomedical evidence has led to a consensus that atherosclerosis is a multifactorial chronic inflammatory disease that starts with the dysfunction of and/or injury to the endothelium, which is the inner lining of artery walls. Although only a single-cell-deep layer, the endothelium regulates the normal functioning of the arterial vessel walls. It acts as the traffic cop responding to the many blood-borne influences and biochemical signals that can modify the arterial walls. When any factor stresses or injures the endothelium, it triggers the inflammatory response that activates a variety of immune system signals and cells that rush to repair the damage.

If this process is triggered just occasionally, then this immune response repairs the damaged cells and shuts down until additional injury occurs. Unfortunately, the damage produced by most risk factors is constant and chronic. Risk factors such as elevated levels of LDL cholesterol and other lipids (fats), high blood pressure, smoking, and insulin resistance and diabetes cause chronic endothelial dysfunction and inflammation, and keep the immune response stuck in the "on" position.

Inflammation serves as a mediator in the disease progression by recruiting various immune system fighter and repair cells. The exact pathways by which inflammation exerts its influence are emerging from current research. Scientists are looking especially for inflammation markers that may help physicians diagnose and treat people at high risk of CHD in its early stages before symptoms arise, when lifestyle and medical therapies may halt or even reverse the disease.

Progressing to fatty streaks

Among the factors causing endothelial dysfunction to progress to atherosclerotic plaque, elevated levels of the certain types of cholesterol, particularly low-density lipoprotein (LDL) cholesterol, and other lipids play a major roll.

Here's an overview of what happens:

1. **Excess LDL cholesterol is deposited on the artery walls.**

   As a basic building block for every cell, cholesterol constantly circulates in the blood along with other substances that are vital for life. When blood levels of cholesterol, particularly LDL cholesterol, are too high, excess LDL cholesterol is deposited on the endothelial lining of arteries where special receptor cells latch on to the LDL molecules.

2. **Trapped LDL damages the cells, triggering the body's immune system into action.**

   This trapped LDL can damage the cells by a process called *oxidation*. The oxidation attracts protective substances related to the immune system. Cells such as macrophages already in artery walls engulf the oxidized excess lipid. (Risk factors also function to create more dangerous LDL particles such as small dense LDL that pass more easily through the endothelial into the first layer of the artery wall, called the *intima*.)

3. **As the immune system tries to remove excess lipids and repair the damage, yellow fatty streaks appear on the artery walls.**

   Soon more circulating fighter cells, known as *monocytes,* enter the artery lining and transform into macrophages to gobble up more excess lipids. Other protective mechanisms such as platelets, T-cells, and growth factors for smooth muscle cells arrive and work hard to restore the damage from excess lipids. As these macrophages engulf the cholesterol, they transform into *macrophage foam cells,* which usually appear as yellow fatty streaks visible on the interior artery walls.

4. **The fatty streaks continue to grow and form scar tissue.**

   When blood cholesterol levels are lower and plenty of HDL cholesterol (the good guys) is present to carry away LDL, then these fatty streaks can be halted or reversed. (For more on cholesterol and controlling it, see Chapter 9.) But when excess cholesterol and/or other risk factors such as the circulating platelets and other clotting factors and excess smooth muscles are present, the deposits typically continue growing. Through pathways not yet clear, risk factors can also help modify HDL lipoproteins so that they no longer act protectively but instead contribute to the atherosclerotic process.

   As the process seals off the excess lipids, it actually creates cholesterol-rich pockets covered with scar tissue. These lesions narrow the arteries and typically deform artery walls as they grow larger.

Growing from fatty streaks to large plaques

Decades of time and the presence of various risk factors are required for the fatty streaks to develop into intermediate (moderate-sized, symptomless) and advanced (larger, symptom-producing) plaques. Figure 2-3 illustrates the typical but gradual development and progression of coronary heart disease.

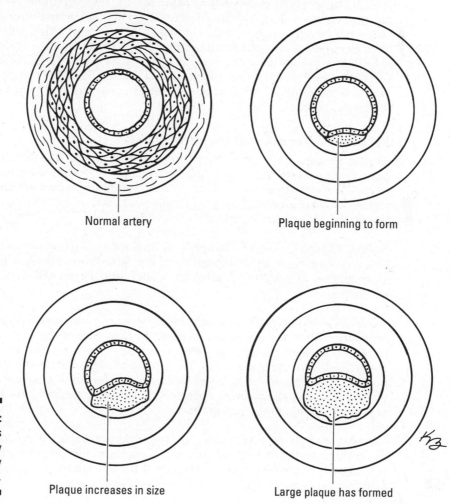

Normal artery

Plaque beginning to form

Plaque increases in size

Large plaque has formed

Figure 2-3:
The process
of coronary
artery
disease.

Illustration by Kathryn Born

Growing to moderate, intermediate types of plaque

In the presence of normal mechanical forces, such as the impact of flowing blood against artery walls, and risk factors that can injure artery walls, many fatty streaks begin growing into larger deposits. More cholesterol and other lipid (fat) particles migrate into the artery walls. This happens particularly in areas where the intima of the artery has thickened, probably to adapt to mechanical forces exerted on the arteries.

More and more fatty substances aren't taken into macrophages or the smooth muscle cells; instead, they begin pooling between them. Some cells die and release their lipids into this core. At that point, a thin layer of intimal tissue has begun forming a cap to contain this lipid pool. Other substances such as *cytokines* (various small proteins active in the immune system) and growth factors may also play a role in forming the cap and helping it continue to grow. The formation and growth of the cap mark the transition from *intermediate* lesions to what medspeak terms *advanced* (and typically more dangerous) *lesions*.

Becoming advanced atherosclerotic plaques

As plaques continue to grow, they reach a condition and size that may produce symptoms such as angina, unstable angina, or even heart attack or stroke. The various advanced types of *atherosclerotic plaques* are characterized by a well-defined lipid core that is contained by a cap composed of layers of smooth muscle cells and other substances.

At first this cap appears to be nearly normal intimal layers. But as the plaque grows larger, the composition of the cap's layers changes, becoming more fibrous, or scarlike, as substances such as collagen and calcium enter the mix.

Some advanced plaques are stable, but others are vulnerable to cracking or rupture. When a crack or tear occurs, the lipid core is exposed to arterial blood from which sticky platelets may trigger the formation of a blood clot intended to repair the break. The clot, however, enlarges the size of the plaque. Some plaques grow larger by a cyclical process of cracking and clotting, which gradually narrows the artery. Fewer plaques may grow by a process of cap erosion rather than rupture.

The plaques that are more vulnerable to cracking are more likely to form a clot that totally blocks the artery and causes a sudden event such as a heart attack or stroke. So looking briefly at the difference between plaques is important — and the topic of the next section.

Differentiating between stable and unstable plaques

As individual plaques grow to moderate size and begin exhibiting the rich lipid core and thin fibrous cap associated with the first level of advanced lesions, they appear to be more vulnerable to rupture and dangerous clot formation than larger, older, thicker plaques. Bigger doesn't necessarily mean more vulnerable, either. The most vulnerable plaques, which can give rise to the deadliest heart attacks, typically block the vessel by only about 40 percent to 50 percent.

Medical scientists and physicians are particularly interested in ways to accurately identify these types of vulnerable plaques, because they seem to be responsible for the majority of sudden acute cardiovascular events, including heart attack, cardiac arrest, and stroke. Figure 2-4 illustrates the way in which such a process suddenly blocks an artery and causes an acute event.

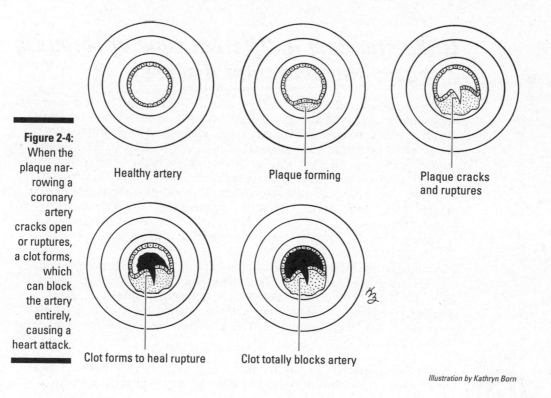

Figure 2-4: When the plaque narrowing a coronary artery cracks open or ruptures, a clot forms, which can block the artery entirely, causing a heart attack.

Healthy artery

Plaque forming

Plaque cracks and ruptures

Clot forms to heal rupture

Clot totally blocks artery

Illustration by Kathryn Born

Current evidence suggests that stable plaques typically have thicker, more fibrous caps with few inflammatory cells and more calcification, which make the cap tougher. Stable plaques also appear to have fewer lipids within. Although stable plaques often are large, the edges or shoulders of the lesion usually are smooth and tapered.

Unstable plaques, by contrast, are smaller in size but are very rich in cholesterol and incorporate many more inflammatory cells, which release chemicals that degrade the fibrous cap. Unstable plaques often appear structurally weak. In addition, the thinner cap may be easily ruptured or torn by a number of forces, ranging from the normal flow of blood at high stress points in the arterial system to sudden pressures such as suddenly increased blood pressure from exertion.

Researchers continue to look for tests and techniques that accurately identify and assess unstable plaque. Such tools would enable physicians to better identify individuals at greater risk of acute events and begin preventive measures.

Understanding a different type of coronary disease: Microvascular disease

Some people who experience reduced flow of blood to the heart do not have narrowings of the larger coronary arteries caused by atherosclerotic plaque. Instead, they have coronary *microvascular disease (MVD)*. MVD occurs much more often in women than men, particularly in premenopausal or younger women. In MVD, smaller blood vessels in the heart, which range from 100 micrometers (about the size of a human hair) to 200 micrometers constrict, preventing adequate oxygenated blood from reaching the heart muscle. As a result, people with MVD may have clear larger coronary arteries but still experience the symptoms of chest pain, although the discomfort is usually more diffuse and may last longer than with angina in CHD.

The causes of MVD are not yet clear, but chronic inflammation appears to play an important role. And the risks factors for CHD, such as high blood pressure (particularly before menopause), unhealthy cholesterol levels, smoking, and diabetes appear to contribute. Current research is also looking for possible risk factors unique to MVD as well as for more effective diagnostic techniques.

If you have symptoms of heart disease (see the next section) but have clear coronary arteries, ask your physician about MVD, particularly if you are a woman.

Knowing when chest pain is an emergency

People with coronary artery disease and angina typically live with this problem for many years and discover how to manage it effectively with appropriate medicines and advice from their physicians. When angina pain changes in character, however, it can signal unstable angina or even heart attack. If you experience any of the following characteristics of chest discomfort, *you need to call 911 and be taken to a hospital immediately:*

✔ Pain or discomfort that is worse than you have ever experienced before

✔ Pain or discomfort that is not relieved by three nitroglycerin tablets in succession, each taken five minutes apart

✔ Pain or discomfort that is accompanied by fainting or lightheadedness, nausea, and/or cool clammy skin

✔ Pain or discomfort lasting longer than 20 minutes

If any of these symptoms occur, you need to call an ambulance and be taken immediately to a hospital. Under no circumstances should you drive yourself to the hospital.

Recognizing the Symptoms and Manifestations of Coronary Heart Disease

Because every person is an individual, physical responses to progressive coronary artery disease vary. Not every individual with heart disease has every manifestation and symptom of the condition. Individuals likewise experience specific symptoms in different ways. But these manifestations are typical:

✔ **Nothing:** Many people can have significant coronary atherosclerosis but experience no discomfort or other sign of the disease. That's why this condition is known in medicine as *silent ischemia. Ischemia* means lack of blood flow. People with diabetes are particularly susceptible to silent ischemia, but others can have it, too.

✔ **Angina:** More formally known as *angina pectoris,* angina is typified by temporary chest pain, usually during exertion. This pain usually is felt as a tightness or uncomfortable feeling across the chest or up to the neck and jaw, not as a sharp stab. Angina also may have other manifestations.

✔ **Unstable angina:** Chest pain that is new, occurs when you're at rest, or suddenly grows more severe is called *unstable angina.* It's a medical emergency.

✔ **Heart attack:** Completely cutting off blood flow to a coronary artery causes an acute heart attack, or *myocardial infarction (MI),* the most severe result of coronary heart disease. The closure can be gradual or the result of a blood clot. A spasm in a coronary artery, particularly in the area of a narrowing, may also result in heart attack.

✔ **Sudden death:** The cause of sudden death from coronary heart disease often is a rhythm problem such as ventricular tachycardia or ventricular fibrillation. These rhythm problems sometimes occur in the setting of an acute heart attack. I've highlighted it here to make the point that the first indication or symptom for some people that they have CHD is a fatal cardiac arrest or heart attack. Many of these deaths happen to people in their 50s, 40s, or younger.

Recognizing angina, or chest pain

Angina typically is a discomfort felt in the chest, often beneath the breastbone (or sternum) or in nearby areas such as the neck, jaw, back, or arms.

✔ Individuals often describe the chest discomfort as a "squeezing sensation," "vicelike," "constricting," or " a heavy pressure on the chest." (In fact, the term *angina* comes from a Greek word that means "strangling" — a strangling pain.)

✔ Angina often is brought on by physical exertion or strong emotions and typically is relieved within several minutes by resting or using nitroglycerin.

✔ Some individuals, particularly women, may experience angina as a symptom different from chest discomfort or in addition to it. Shortness of breath, nausea, faintness, abdominal pain, indigestion, or extreme fatigue may also be manifestations of angina.

✔ When chest pain occurs at rest, it usually is classified as *unstable angina.*

And just how do you pronounce the word? Some people say "an-*jī*-nuh" and others say "*an*-juh-nuh." Either is correct. Some cardiologists may be a little snobby about their preference (who, us?), but pay them no mind.

Understanding the causes of angina

You know how your muscles begin to scream when you run faster than your blood can carry adequate oxygen to them. The same thing may happen when the coronary arteries become so narrowed by atherosclerotic plaques that blood flow to the heart is inadequate to supply the heart muscle with the oxygen it needs. The temporary chest discomfort known as *angina* is your heart's way of getting your attention. It occurs when you ask your heart to work harder, and it therefore demands more blood — for instance, when you're walking briskly or running, climbing a hill or stairs, having sex, or doing housework or yardwork. Strong emotions such as fear or anger also can trigger an episode.

Considering angina's effect on the heart

Angina usually does not damage the heart. It is a temporary condition — the usual episode lasts only 5 to 10 minutes. (In MVD, the episodes can last longer, about 10 minutes up to 30 minutes.) Chest discomfort makes you stop and rest, slowing the heart and lessening its demand for blood. Alternatively, most people with angina know to take a nitroglycerin tablet under the tongue when they have an angina attack. The nitroglycerin dilates the coronary arteries, enabling blood flow to the heart to increase.

Any discomfort that doesn't stop with rest or that lasts more than 5 to 10 minutes may be a heart attack and needs to be treated as an emergency.

Diagnosing angina

An individual's own description of the discomfort he or she experiences provides the most important information leading to the diagnosis of angina. However, your physician will typically order appropriate tests based on your symptoms and signs. These may range from an electrocardiogram, exercise stress test, or stress echocardiogram to nuclear stress testing and cardiac catheterization (see Chapter 13). Some of these tests can be conducted in your physician's office, but others require the resources of a hospital.

Distinguishing other causes of chest pain

All chest pain is not angina and does not involve the heart. Various conditions involving other structures in the chest can occasionally cause chest discomfort; these include spasm of the esophagus, acid reflux, hiatal hernia, and muscular pain.

Treating angina

People who have angina typically can live comfortably for many years with this condition by finding out how to manage the symptoms and lower their risk factors for complications.

Developing angina can be a big blow emotionally. So big that patients often adopt an unrealistically gloomy perception of their prognosis. Actually, there's much you can do to adapt. Start with an open, frank discussion with your physician about the following lifestyle modifications:

- ✔ Adjusting your approach to physical activity, leisure-time pursuits, eating habits, and other practices to reduce risk factors and control and even reduce the symptoms of angina.

- ✔ Modifying strenuous activities that consistently and repeatedly produce angina, by taking simple measures such as slowing your walking pace, strolling (not sprinting) to the car through the rain, vacuuming or raking more slowly, and so on.

- ✔ Avoiding strenuous activities that require heavy lifting, such as snow shoveling (unless you discuss it with your physician).

- ✔ Adding slowly progressive exercise training, under your physician's supervision, which can dramatically increase your ability to perform enjoyable activities of daily living.

- ✔ Considering with your physician other interventions such as medication or surgery if your angina causes unacceptably severe modifications of your lifestyle because quality of life is important!

Defining Unstable Angina

As the name suggests, *unstable angina* results when angina gets out of control. In unstable angina, the lack of blood flow and oxygen to the heart becomes acute and, therefore, very dangerous because the risk of complications such as heart attack is much greater.

Where stable angina has typical characteristics and predictable triggers, such as exertion or strong emotion, unstable angina is characterized by one or more of the following symptoms:

- ✔ Anginal discomfort at rest or when awakening from sleep

- ✔ A significant change in the pattern of the angina where it occurs with less exertion or is more severe than before

- ✔ A significant increase in the severity or frequency of angina

- ✔ New onset, or first experience, of anginal chest pain

If you experience any one of these characteristics, you must seek immediate medical attention.

Defining a Heart Attack

A heart attack, known medically as a *myocardial infarction (MI),* occurs when one of the three coronary arteries that supply oxygen-rich blood to the heart muscle *(myocardium)* becomes severely or totally blocked, usually by a blood clot. When the heart muscle doesn't receive enough oxygenated blood, it begins to die. The severity of the heart attack depends on how much of the heart is injured or dies when the attack occurs.

When you think you're having a heart attack it's critical to go immediately to a hospital by ambulance where therapy can be initiated to save your heart muscle from dying. New clot-busting medicines, as well as procedures such as angioplasty, often can dissolve a clot that causes the heart attack, open the blood vessel, and save some or all of the heart muscle at risk. Although some of the heart muscle usually dies during a heart attack, the remaining heart muscle continues to function and often can compensate, to a very large degree, for the heart muscle that has died.

Understanding the causes of a heart attack

Heart attack almost always is caused when a blood clot forms at the site of an existing fatty plaque that has narrowed the coronary artery. Thus, individuals are at much higher risk for heart attack if they

- ✔ Have a history of coronary heart disease
- ✔ Have experienced previous bouts of angina
- ✔ Have suffered a previous heart attack

The blockage that triggers a heart attack usually is caused by an acute blood clot. Most *acute blood clots* occur when one of the plaques or fatty deposits on the artery walls cracks or ruptures. Other, much more rare causes of acute blockages in arteries, such as a severe coronary artery spasm, can also cause heart attack.

Recognizing the symptoms of a heart attack

Different people experience the symptoms of a heart attack in different ways. However, typical symptoms include some or all of the following symptoms (as described by the American Heart Association):

- ✔ Uncomfortable pressure, fullness, squeezing, or pain in the center of the chest lasting more than a few minutes
- ✔ Pain spreading to the shoulders, neck, or arms
- ✔ Chest discomfort with lightheadedness, fainting, sweating, nausea, or shortness of breath

In an individual who has angina, symptoms may be particularly difficult to differentiate from the chest discomfort of angina. However, when a heart attack is occurring, chest discomfort usually is more severe and may occur while the individual is at rest or less active than usual.

The signs of a heart attack often are subtle, particularly with individuals who have diabetes. People with diabetes may not have the classic symptoms of chest, shoulder, or arm discomfort. Chest pain experienced by many women likewise may not present the classic symptoms.

 Coronary heart disease (CHD) is extremely common in men and women in the United States and particularly in men in their 40s and older and postmenopausal women. Even if you've never had a single sign of trouble, you need to call 911 and go straight to the hospital for prompt evaluation whenever you experience any of the preceding warning signs. Do not take a meeting. Do not put it off for an hour . . . *just call 911 and go!*

 About two-thirds of the individuals who experience an acute heart attack also experience some warning symptoms in the weeks or days preceding the acute event. They often don't realize what the warning signs were until after the event — with keen hindsight. So work on your foresight. That way you'll know the warning signs of heart attack and take them seriously.

Differentiating between heart attack and sudden cardiac arrest

 Although doctors often call sudden cardiac arrest "a massive heart attack," the two technically are not the same thing. A *massive heart attack* (myocardial infarction) results from a blockage of the coronary arteries. *Sudden cardiac arrest* is caused by ventricular fibrillation, an electrical malfunction in which the heart begins to quiver rapidly, instead of contracting and pumping blood regularly. Cardiac arrest strikes without warning. Because blood flow essentially stops, victims of cardiac arrest lose consciousness and die within minutes unless emergency help is available.

Many victims of sudden cardiac arrest have underlying CHD. Sudden cardiac arrest often (but not always) occurs in the setting of an acute heart attack. It can also occur from electrical malfunction when a heart attack is not involved.

Taking Action — Immediately — for a Possible Heart Attack

Unfortunately, many people who are experiencing a heart attack either don't recognize symptoms or deny them. Doing so can be a serious or even fatal mistake, because delay

✔ Significantly increases the risk of sudden death from heart rhythm problems in the early phases of a heart attack.

✔ Increases the likelihood that a significant amount of heart muscle will die, thus increasing the likelihood and extent of the heart attack, causing disability if the individual survives.

Timing is everything! If you or a loved one experiences any symptoms or warning signs of a heart attack, use the six-point survival plan I outline here in the following points. Don't delay!

This six-point survival plan, adapted from American Medical Association recommendations, can save your life. Take these steps if you or a loved one is experiencing the symptoms of a possible heart attack:

1. **Stop what you are doing, and sit or lie down.**

2. **If symptoms persist for more than two minutes, call your local emergency number or 911 and say that you may be having a heart attack.**

   Leave the phone off the hook so that medical personnel can locate your address in the event that you become unconscious.

3. **Take nitroglycerin, if possible.**

   If you have nitroglycerin tablets, take up to three pills under your tongue, one at a time, every five minutes, if your chest pain persists.

   If you don't have nitroglycerin, take two aspirin.

4. **Do not drive yourself (or a loved one) to the hospital if you think you are having a heart attack.**

   Ambulances have equipment and personnel who are trained to deal with individuals who are having a heart attack. Driving yourself or a loved one to the hospital is an invitation for a disaster.

5. **If the person's pulse or breathing stops, any individual trained in cardiopulmonary resuscitation (CPR) needs to immediately begin to administer it.**

   If an automated external defibrillator (AED) is available, use it. Call 911 immediately, but do not delay instituting CPR or using an AED.

6. **When you arrive at the hospital emergency room, announce clearly that you (or your loved one) may be having a heart attack and that you must be seen immediately.**

    Don't be shy about it.

Other Manifestations of Heart Disease

Atherosclerosis, angina, and heart attack aren't the only types of heart disease. This section looks briefly at four other common types of heart disease — arrhythmias (rhythm problems), heart failure, stroke, and heart valve problems.

Arrhythmias

Arrhythmias (or *dysrhythmias*) refer to problems with the electrical system that controls the heart's normal rhythm. They may occur in the context of an acute heart attack or from other causes.

When the electrical system goes entirely haywire, it may result in a very dangerous condition called *ventricular tachycardia,* which occurs when an abnormal electrical impulse causes the heart to beat so fast that it cannot pump out adequate blood. This condition can rapidly degenerate to *ventricular fibrillation,* which occurs when the heart simply quivers and produces no blood flow. Ventricular fibrillation must be immediately terminated by an electrical shock, or *defibrillation,* administered by a medical professional.

The *atria,* the upper chambers that assist the ventricles (refer to Figure 2-1), can also have rhythm problems. One of the most common is *atrial fibrillation. Atrial fibrillation* occurs when electrical signals are chaotic, and muscles of the atria quiver rather than contract. The electrical impulses also reach the ventricles very erratically, thus producing an erratic heartbeat. This condition is common in individuals who have heart disease and can be caused by a variety of conditions including coronary heart disease, hypertension, and an elevated thyroid level.

Atrial fibrillation, by itself, is not immediately life-threatening. But because the atria are not contracting effectively, they can gather clots that can pass through the heart and into either the brain, potentially resulting in a stroke, or the lungs, potentially resulting in a very serious condition called *pulmonary embolism.* Because of the possible outcomes, treating atrial fibrillation aggressively is important. Treatment may include medications and/or *cardioversion* (an electrical procedure that restores normal rhythms). In addition to medicines to control the heart rate, all patients who have atrial fibrillation must take blood-thinning medicines (anticoagulants) to lower the risk of blood clots generated in the atria being thrown to the brain or lungs.

Heart failure

Heart failure occurs when the heart no longer adequately pumps blood to the lungs and throughout the body. It usually is a slow process that takes place during a period of years. Underlying conditions, such as CHD, leakage from one of the heart valves, an acute heart attack, or various diseases of the heart muscle itself usually cause heart failure.

The heart initially compensates for small decreases in its ability to pump by doing the following:

✔ Enlarging *(dilatation)* to enable more blood into its pumping chambers

✔ Thickening the muscle walls *(hypertrophy)* to strengthen the pump and enable it to exert more force during its contraction to move more blood

✔ Beating faster to make up for decreased volume or power (like trying to pitch more, but smaller, pails of water on a fire)

The heart may try to compensate in these ways for years before you notice any symptoms. But when these mechanisms ultimately fail, significant heart failure occurs. By then, compensatory mechanisms often have become part of the problem.

How serious heart failure is depends on how much pumping capacity the heart has lost. A normal heart discharges about 60 to 75 percent of the blood in the main pumping chambers with each contraction, or beat. Heart failure often occurs when the amount of blood ejected per beat, called the *ejection fraction,* drops below 50 percent, and when the ejection fraction falls below 40 percent heart failure ensues. Even so, many people can survive for many years with ejection fractions of only 20 to 30 percent, or sometimes even 15 percent.

All forms of heart failure are serious health problems that require medical treatment. Taking care of yourself, seeing your physician regularly, and paying scrupulous attention to recommended treatments including lifestyle modifications are important steps you can take to improve your chances of living longer. Fortunately, many effective treatments are now available for heart failure and experimental procedures such as stem cell therapy are promising.

Stroke

A stroke occurs when a blood clot or bleeding suddenly interrupts the flow of blood to an area of the brain. When deprived of blood, brain cells lose their ability to function and, if deprived for too long, die. Because brain cells and groups of brain cells have highly specialized functions, the location of stroke damage determines what loss of neurological and bodily function occurs as a result of stroke. Impairment may be temporary or permanent.

Strokes are categorized in two basic ways: ischemic stroke and hemorrhagic stroke. The causes and results of stroke depend on how and where the stroke occurs.

Ischemic stroke

An ischemic stroke occurs when a blood clot or other particle blocks a blood vessel in the brain and cuts off the blood supply to the portion of the brain supplied by that vessel. Without adequate oxygen, that portion of the brain suffers damage or even dies. This type of stroke is called an *ischemic stroke* because it's caused by *ischemia,* the medical term for lack of blood flow.

About 70 to 80 percent of all strokes are ischemic, and they occur in two basic forms:

✔ **Cerebral thrombosis:** This form of stroke results from progressive narrowing of arteries in the brain or sometimes in the carotid arteries in the neck. In a thrombosis, plaque (there's that cholesterol again) that narrows the artery and any clot *(thrombus)* that forms on it doesn't move, meaning the typical underlying causes for this type of blockage are atherosclerosis and high blood pressure. Before having a major stroke, many people experience a temporary lack of blood flow to the brain that's called a *transient ischemic attack* (TIA), which actually is a small stroke in which the effects usually last for only a few minutes or hours.

Never ignore possible TIA symptoms; treat them as a serious warning and consult your physician.

✔ **Cerebral embolism:** This form of stroke occurs when a blood clot, or *embolus,* travels from somewhere else in the body to the brain. When the blood clot lodges in a vessel in the brain, it cuts off blood flow to the portion of the brain supplied by that vessel. Blood clots that cause strokes may form in and travel from a number of different locations in the body, including:

• **Major arteries in the neck that supply the brain (the carotid arteries).** This is why your doctor often listens with a stethoscope over your neck to hear whether any narrowing of one of these arteries has occurred. The narrowing of the artery leads to turbulence that the doctor can hear.

• **The heart — particularly in people with atrial fibrillation.** In this case, when the upper chambers, or atria, fibrillate instead of contracting normally, blood clots can form in the blood and travel directly from the left atrium to the brain.

Hemorrhagic stroke

A hemorrhagic stroke occurs when a blood vessel in or on the brain bursts and bleeds into the brain or into the space between the brain and skull. This type of stroke is called a hemorrhagic stroke because it's caused by a *hemorrhage* (in Greek, *hemo* means "blood" and *rhage* means "to break"). The brain is very sensitive to bleeding and pressure, which damage brain tissue, often permanently. Hemorrhagic strokes account for only about 20 percent of all strokes, but they usually are more severe and more often fatal than ischemic stroke.

Heart valve problems

As I discuss earlier in this chapter, the four heart valves serve as traffic cops of the heart, directing blood flow in the proper direction and preventing it from improperly backing up.

As long as these valves open fully and shut tightly, all is well. But if any disease or injury causes valve leakage *(regurgitation)* or narrowing *(stenosis)*, major problems can result. Significant valve leakage can overload the heart because extra blood flowing back into the heart requires an extra strong beat to eject it. A narrowed valve can cause the heart to thicken because it is being asked to pump against a much higher pressure.

A number of different conditions cause valves to leak or narrow, including:

- Congenital valvular problems (a condition you're born with).
- Damage to valve structures, such as when the structures that anchor the flaps of the mitral valve break. Heart attack can also seriously damage the muscles that control the valves.
- Progressive problems, including those that may result from the aging process, such as calcification, or those that result from an infection, such as rheumatic fever or endocarditis. If the problem becomes too severe, it may require open-heart surgery and valve replacement.

If a valve abnormality is not progressing rapidly or causing any serious problem, your physician may simply keep a close eye on it so that treatment can be initiated when and if it becomes necessary. Following a heart-healthy diet and lifestyle can also support valve health. Taking preventive antibiotics as needed when you have an underlying valve abnormality is a good idea. There are also various medical and surgical treatments for valve problems.

Chapter 3

Are You at Risk of Heart Disease? How to Turn That Risk Around

*H*eart disease takes many forms, and established and emerging risk factors contribute to each form of heart disease in complex ways. In this chapter, I discuss the risk factors for *atherosclerosis,* particularly in the context of coronary heart disease (CHD). Paying close attention to the roles the various risk factors play and taking steps to control them can go a long way toward slowing or even reversing heart disease.

Defining Risk Factors

What is a risk factor anyway? Just as the name suggests, a *risk factor* is something that increases your chances of developing a chronic condition — that is, an ongoing health condition that you must live with. In the case of cardiac health, a risk factor is a personal habit, practice, or physical characteristic or condition that increases the likelihood that you'll develop heart disease. In other words, risk factors contribute to the progression of the disease or condition.

Scientific research is continuously revealing more about the risk factors for developing atherosclerosis, particularly coronary heart disease. Our basic understanding has grown primarily through a number of long-term studies of very large groups. The foundational study is the Framingham Heart Study, which has followed in great detail the lifestyle and health records of more than 5,000 men and women since 1948 and another group of more than 5,000 of their children since 1971.

Over time, findings from this study and many other large population studies and clinical trials have identified a number of risk factors that independently, directly, and significantly increase your risk of developing heart disease. Research has also identified additional factors that contribute to cardiovascular disease risks or that may serve as biomarkers that doctors may be able to use to better diagnose atherosclerosis in earlier stages of the disease and/or when it occurs in people who have no risk factors or no symptoms.

Identifying important risk factors

For many years, risk factors that directly and significantly affected heart health were called *major risk factors.* Today, with the constant outpouring of new research findings about potential risks and biomarkers, such established risk factors are more typically called *traditional risk factors.* Other established factors that do not, according to the current research data, demonstrate as direct an impact may be called *contributing risk factors.* In addition to these established risk factors, extensive ongoing research regularly identifies and refines understanding of factors or markers related to heart health that are usually called *emerging, nontraditional,* or *novel* risk factors or biomarkers. These last also include exploration of promising genetic links to heart disease.

Sounds fairly complex, right? I'd agree — the stream of new research can be confusing. However, you should remember that extensive evidence supports the importance of the major traditional risk factors. Newer research typically refines and expands our understanding of the mechanisms and markers behind how these risk factors work.

Most usefully, you can divide the primary risk factors into those that you can change and those you can't (though you should be aware of how the latter interact with risks you can modify). Important risk factors you can change for the better though lifestyle practices include smoking, unhealthy cholesterol levels, high blood pressure, physical activity, obesity, and diabetes. Those you can't modify include advancing age, your gender, and a family history of premature heart disease. I discuss each of these risk factors and promising emerging factors and biomarkers in this chapter.

Multiplying risks — double trouble and more

One aspect of risk factors that makes them particularly dangerous is that their effects multiply, rather than merely add up, whenever you exhibit two or more of them. If you have only a single major risk factor, you typically double your chance of developing heart disease. When two risk factors are present, the possibility quadruples. And, worse yet, when three risk factors join forces, the possibility of your developing heart disease increases 8 to 20 times! If you think that's bad news, listen to this: Having two and three risk factors is not unusual. In fact, risk factors have a distinct tendency to occur in clusters, particularly in the presence of obesity or diabetes.

Heading off trouble by controlling risk

Ideally, you would have no lifestyle-related risks for heart disease. If you are a young adult or for your young children, this may actually be true. In that case, your goal should be to adopt lifestyle practices that preserve such ideal heart health. In medicine, this is sometimes called *primordial prevention*. (No, you aren't heading back to the dawn of all time, but just maintaining the presumably ideal health you had as a newborn — the dawn of your life.)

How can you usefully measure such ideal heart health? The American Heart Association in setting cardiovascular health goals for 2020 identified seven health behaviors and measures that defined ideal cardiovascular health:

- Not smoking
- Maintaining a healthy weight (indicated by body mass index)
- Being physically active at recommended levels
- Achieving a healthy diet score
- Maintaining total cholesterol below 200 mg/dL (untreated)
- Maintaining blood pressure in the neighborhood of 120/80 mg/dL (untreated or treated)
- Fasting blood glucose of less than 100 mg/dL (untreated)

Do you meet all seven of these criteria or do you join most American adults? At the time of the report, less than 5 percent of U.S. adults met all seven criteria. Recent surveys of heart health show little improvement. So the chances are high that you have at least one or more habits or conditions that put you at risk of developing heart disease sometime in the future.

Here's the good news. For most risk factors, including these seven, what you helped create you can also change by adopting healthful lifestyle practices. The same is true for the rest of the family, including your children. I show you how to go about that in Parts II and III of this book. If you have one or more risk factors now, no matter how healthy you feel, your goal should be to reduce and control them in order to prevent developing any manifestations of heart disease such as angina or a heart attack. This is called *primary prevention* in medspeak.

If you already have heart disease or have experienced a heart event, such as angina or a heart attack, attempting to bring these same factors under control usually decreases your risk of having further complications and manifestations of heart disease. Actively working toward this goal with the support of your doctor and healthcare team is called *secondary prevention.* (See Chapter 15 for tips about taking back your life after you have heart disease or a heart event.)

Tailoring prevention to individual needs

Controlling or treating a particular risk factor may mean different things for different individuals. One size does not fit all. For example, a young woman with a mildly elevated total cholesterol level — say 215 mg/dl — but no other risk factors may require only healthful modifications in diet and physical activity. On the other hand, a 60-year-old man who's already suffered a heart attack and has the same level of elevated cholesterol may require immediate, aggressive treatment to lower his cholesterol levels. (See Chapter 9 for more about cholesterol.)

Because a young woman with an elevated cholesterol level has a relatively greater risk of developing coronary heart disease than a young woman who doesn't have an elevated cholesterol level, she needs to work with her physician on modifying lifestyle habits to lower her cholesterol. Her situation is not as immediately threatening and therefore doesn't need to be treated as aggressively as that of the 60-year-old man with heart disease and elevated cholesterol. Because his elevated cholesterol comes in the context of existing heart disease, therapy for him needs to be much more intensive. In treating heart disease, controlling risk factors is an important part of every treatment regimen.

Tackling Risk Factors That You Can Control

If you have any of the following risk factors related to lifestyle, you can significantly cut your risks of ever developing heart disease. If you already have silent signs of atherosclerosis, such as some plaque in your coronary arteries, in many instances, taking steps to aggressively control these risk factors may even help reverse or at least halt the disease process.

Having hypertension — high blood pressure

Landmark studies conducted in the 1960s put to rest any serious doubt that elevated blood pressure, or *hypertension,* represents a substantial risk for developing CHD and stroke. Hypertension appears to be particularly dangerous in terms of the likelihood of developing a stroke. (For an in-depth discussion of hypertension, see Chapter 8.)

Hypertension is extremely common in the United States, probably because of the nutritional habits, propensity to gain weight, and sedentary lifestyle of most Americans. More than a third of the entire adult population in the United States suffers from hypertension. By the time an individual reaches age 60, he or she has a greater than 65 percent chance of having elevated blood pressure. About 20 percent of people with high blood pressure don't know they have it — no wonder it's called the *silent killer.*

Once again, the good news is that daily habits and practices, such as appropriate weight control, sound nutrition, and regular physical activity, can profoundly diminish the likelihood of your ever developing hypertension in the first place and can significantly contribute to the effective treatment of elevated blood pressure. (For more about these healthful practices, see Chapters 5 and 10.) In fact, controlling blood pressure within normal levels is an important part of both primary and secondary prevention of heart disease (and kidney disease, the other great health risk of hypertension).

Having unhealthy cholesterol levels

By now, almost everyone knows having a high total cholesterol level in your blood is a bad thing. When it comes to being at risk of developing CHD, however, an elevated level of blood cholesterol is only one of a number of *lipid problems* (problems with fats in the blood) that significantly elevate your risk of heart disease. The abnormalities that are particularly dangerous include elevated total cholesterol, elevated LDL cholesterol, low HDL cholesterol, elevated triglycerides, or any combination of the four.

The good news is that by following appropriate lifestyle measures and, in some instances, using the effective medicines that now are available, you can manage this risk factor for coronary heart disease. You can get all the definitions, evidence, and strategies for better controlling cholesterol levels in Chapter 9.

Using tobacco

Cigarette smoking (and the use of other tobacco products) is the leading cause of premature death in the United States each year, claiming more than 450,000 lives.

Although cigarette smoking has declined, unfortunately about 21 percent of adult men and 16 percent of adult women still smoke cigarettes. Shockingly, although many adults successfully struggle to quit cigarette smoking, an estimated 6,400 children start smoking every day.

The health consequences of cigarette smoking are severe. Smoking

- ✔ Triples the risk of developing heart disease and increases the risk of developing lung cancer by a whopping 3,000 percent.

- ✔ Increases the risk of harming the health of others. Individuals with CHD can have angina attacks provoked merely by being in a smoke-filled room.

- ✔ Tends to lower HDL cholesterol (the good guys).

In an otherwise bleak picture, the outstanding good news is that stopping smoking

- ✔ Lowers the risk of developing coronary heart disease and significantly improves the health outlook for individuals who have heart disease.

- ✔ Improves blood lipids. In one study, LDL cholesterol decreased more than 5 percent, and HDL cholesterol increased more than 3 percent in individuals who stopped cigarette smoking.

Quitting is so important (and so tough) that Chapter 11 is devoted to the facts and strategies you need so that you can find the ways and means and support to stamp out smoking in your life.

Being physically inactive

Physical inactivity results first in a lack of cardiac fitness. That means your deconditioned heart demands more oxygen and has to pump faster to do its job. Getting just 150 minutes of moderate activity weekly or 75 minutes of intensive activity can turn that ugly picture around. Physical activity directly supports heart health by helping to lower inflammation, improve your lipid profile, lower blood pressure, and improve insulin sensitivity and endothelial function. (The endothelium is the inner lining of the arteries; refer to Chapter 2 for details.)

As you can see, physical activity is important to heart health not just because it increases cardiac fitness but because it can contribute significantly to controlling other major risk factors, such as high blood pressure, elevated blood cholesterol, diabetes, and obesity.

If you are currently inactive or mostly sedentary, it's not hard to turn this sad picture around. You can get off your duff and start by accumulating two or three five-minute walks a day and build up from there. (See Chapter 5 for help.) In addition to reducing your risks of heart disease and its contributing conditions, regular physical active will also help you look *good* and feel *better*.

Being obese or overweight

Like physical inactivity, obesity and overweight also contribute to many other risk factors, including hypertension and elevated cholesterol and other abnormal lipid levels. Obesity also puts you at risk for diabetes, another dangerous risk factor.

Unfortunately, for the last few years, the prevalence of obesity and overweight among U.S. adults has held steady at about 66 percent, according to the Centers for Disease Control. More than one in every three adults is now considered obese. By *obese,* I mean weighing at least 20 percent more than desirable body weight. That's not as fat as most people think, either. For example, if your optimal weight is 150 pounds and you weigh 180 — just 30 pounds overweight — you are technically obese even if you think you still look pretty good. Another third of adults are overweight, which also poses increased risks.

Carrying extra weight around the abdomen (sometimes called *abdominal obesity* or *apple-shaped obesity*) is particularly dangerous in terms of its risk of coronary heart disease. Overweight individuals, who, in addition to excess weight, often face one or more other risk factors for heart disease, are particularly susceptible to dying from heart disease because of probable abnormalities caused by fat cells in general and abdominal fat cells in particular.

If you're overweight, regardless of whether you have heart disease, you need to make a point of talking to your doctor about whether you show signs of having other risk factors for heart disease in addition to obesity. The odds are that you do.

Weight loss in and of itself is a highly effective way of reducing multiple risk factors for heart disease. Losing as little as 10 to 15 pounds, or 5 to 10 percent of your weight, can significantly improve matters. A weight management plan that includes both regular physical activity and a reduced-energy but nutrient rich diet can help you succeed. In Chapter 10, I discuss effective weight management principles and strategies and how to create a lifestyle plan to achieve your weight management goals. Chapter 5 covers the basics of achieving healthful nutrition and developing an effective activity program. If you've been diagnosed with heart disease and are overweight, then be sure to discuss these issues with your physician.

Remember, obese people do not die because they are too fat; they die of heart disease.

Having diabetes mellitus

Approximately 29 million adults in the United States, or 9.3 percent of the population, suffer from diabetes mellitus. These figures represent an increase of over 10 million (an increase of 3 percent of the population) in about a decade. Among adults age 65 and older, about 26 percent have diabetes. Another 37 percent of adults (51 percent of those 65 and older) have prediabetes, which is characterized by insulin insensitivity or glucose intolerance.

About 90 to 95 percent of these individuals have type 2 diabetes, which is closely associated with lifestyle-related practices. The rate of type 2 diabetes is also increasing in children and youth. Diabetes represents a significant risk factor for coronary heart disease. In fact, coronary heart disease is by far the leading cause of death in individuals with diabetes.

Individuals with diabetes often have multiple blood lipid abnormalities including elevated blood triglycerides, elevated LDL cholesterol, and depressed HDL cholesterol. Having this particular constellation of lipid abnormalities spells triple trouble! For reasons that to date are not totally clear, women with diabetes have an even greater risk of developing heart disease than men with diabetes.

By working with your physician if you have diabetes, however, you can lower many of the complications of diabetes and also control your blood lipids. Daily steps that you can take to help you control diabetes include weight loss if you're overweight, regular physical activity, and proper nutritional habits.

Experiencing stress and/or depression

Without a doubt, physical and emotional linkages exist between the mind and the heart.

Research evidence increasingly suggests that an individual's response to acute and chronic stress from various environmental pressures and psychosocial factors, such as isolation, anger, and depression, may contribute to heart disease. For example, individuals who exhibit Type A behaviors — people who persistently are rushed and unhappy and particularly those who face the world with high levels of hostility — are at increased risk for developing heart disease. Research suggests that these negative psychological states may influence negative behaviors, such as eating poorly or overeating and being sedentary, which contribute to other risk factors. In addition, stress, depression, and other such emotions may actually trigger some physiological processes that affect the build up of atherosclerotic plaque in the arteries or influence clot formation.

Much promising research into the effects of stress on heart disease is underway. Meanwhile, the potential risks of stress and benefits of properly addressing it are clear enough, and if you experience high levels of stress in your life, exploring ways of lowering it is worthwhile. See Chapter 6 for strategies.

Watching for Risk Factors That You Cannot Modify

Now I come to three risk factors that you can't modify: your age, gender, and family history. Having one or more of these nonmodifiable risk factors makes it particularly important that you pay close attention to the risk factors that you *can* modify:

- ✔ **Age:** Age is considered a significant risk factor for heart disease for men who are older than 45 and for women who are older than 55 or have undergone premature menopause.

- ✔ **Gender:** Men are more likely to develop coronary heart disease than women. Furthermore, the onset of symptoms typically occurs ten years later in women than in men; however, pointing out that heart disease remains the number-one killer in *both* men and women in the United States is important. It becomes particularly prevalent in women after menopause. After age 65, men and women have approximately the same risk for developing CHD.

- ✔ **Family history and heredity:** Heart disease tends to occur more frequently in some families than in others. Coming from a family in which premature coronary heart disease has occurred significantly increases your risk of developing CHD. By *premature coronary heart disease* I mean a diagnosed heart condition or the experience of a heart attack or other heart even before age 55 in males or age 65 in females. Having a first-degree relative (father, mother, brother, or sister) who fits this description qualifies as a risk factor. The likelihood of having cholesterol or lipid disorders may also run in some families; this condition requires working closely with your doctor starting as early as possible to reduce risk.

Paying Attention to Emerging Risk Factors

Research continues to identify factors that may increase or decrease your risk for developing CHD. Among the many potential factors being researched, the following potential risks factors illustrate the type of inquiries. Because the following have received considerable media attention, discussing them with your physician may be worthwhile:

✔ **Homocysteine:** *Homocysteine* is an amino acid that serves as a building block of proteins in the body. However, some studies show that elevated concentrations of homocysteine in the blood can be associated with increased risk of CHD. Currently, research also focuses on other chronic diseases for which homocysteine may be a marker. Fortunately, relatively simple measures, in particular making sure that your diet contains foods rich in *folic acid* (also referred to as *folate*), can reduce elevated levels of homocysteine. The recommended daily value is 400 micrograms of folate per day. Good food sources of folic acid include fruits, green leafy vegetables, tomatoes, whole grains, and low-fat dairy.

Although daily consumption of 400 mcg of folic acid may be a reasonable health decision where the risk of developing heart disease is concerned, it is absolutely mandatory for women of childbearing age, because it helps prevent birth defects related to brain and spine development, including spina bifida. Discuss this issue with your doctor.

✔ **Low levels of antioxidants in the blood:** In recent years, antioxidants have been hyped by the popular media as the cure *du jour* for several conditions, including risk of heart disease. Several studies have supported the concept that low levels of antioxidants in blood may increase the risk of developing CHD. These findings have led to clinical trials of supplementary antioxidants such as vitamin E, vitamin C, and/or beta-carotene (vitamin A). Results of trials to date do not confirm any benefit for supplementation of vitamins E and C, and some findings indicate potential harm from beta-carotene supplementation. Current advice is to turn first to whole foods as the best source for antioxidants and to discuss the issue with your doctor about what is right for you.

✔ **Abnormal blood clotting:** Substantial evidence has emerged indicating that how your blood clots is part of the process of acute coronary heart disease. Certain rare clotting abnormalities clearly increase the risk of coronary heart disease for some individuals. But at this time, using blood-clotting parameters to determine an individual's risk of developing heart disease is highly experimental. If you have questions about whether this rare problem relates to you, discuss it with your physician.

✔ **Markers or factors for specific heart conditions:** Beyond continuing research on the contribution of major risk factors to heart disease, some of the most promising current research concerns identifying specific *markers,* or factors that may indicate an increased risk of developing a specific condition or event. In addition to discovering how such markers work physically, researchers are exploring the potential clinical use of such markers to help diagnose and treat patients. The following examples give you an idea of the nature and promise of such research:

- **Elevated C-Reactive Protein:** Elevated blood levels of *C-Reactive Protein (CRP),* a marker that increases during systemic inflammation (inflammation that affects the whole body), are associated with increased heart attacks and other heart events caused by blood clots. Studies consistently show that higher levels of CRP predict a higher risk of heart attack.

  High CRP is associated with the increased occurrence of new heart events and a lower survival rate in individuals who have unstable angina or have had a heart attack. CRP may also prove useful in predicting a higher risk of heart attack for healthy individuals who don't have elevated cholesterol or CHD symptoms.

  In addition to broadening the populations studied beyond men and women of European heritage, ongoing research continues to explore ways in which CRP levels may provide indicators that are useful in preventing, diagnosing, and treating various manifestations of cardiovascular disease.

- **Lp(a) cholesterol:** This genetic variation of LDL cholesterol (the bad guys) is clearly associated with a greater risk of prematurely developing CHD. Research into how this marker may be useful diagnostically is one aspect of ongoing research.

- **Factor V Leiden:** About 2 to 7 percent of persons of European descent have this variation of the factor V gene, a variant that promotes the formation of blood clots in blood vessels. Persons with V Leiden are at greater risk of developing heart attack, stroke, and deep vein thrombosis. But risk among individuals with this variant appears to vary widely. Current research into gene modifiers is exploring ways to accurately identify individuals who are at greatest risk.

Part II
Taking Basic Steps to Heart Health

Five Ways to Engage the Family in Heart-Healthy Eating and Activity

- ✔ Eat dinner together as a family. Eating dinner together daily or on as many nights as possible improves nutrient intakes for children and adults. Dining together also gives families time to share and communicate, which improves everyone's sense of well-being.

- ✔ Set an example of healthy behaviors for your children. Children learn good habits from parents who eat in healthful ways and who are active. Don't just model good activities; do them together as a family.

- ✔ Engage in family activities two or three times a week. Take a walk as a family after dinner whenever you can. Plan a weekly activity outing — a hike, a trip to a museum or zoo that requires walking, or a outdoor weekend at a state park.

- ✔ Involve children in meal planning and preparation. Children and teens who help plan healthy meals, help shop for the ingredients, and help prepare the meals are most like to develop healthy eating habits. Plus, they'll know how to shop and cook when they leave the nest.

- ✔ Enjoy a regular family game and story night. The first rule is no screens. Haul out the board games. Don't forget party games like charades. Tell stories — family history, funny events, jokes, and interesting events from the past week. Laugh! Physically and emotionally, family night will do your heart good.

See how to use your body mass index (BMI) to motivate your weight loss at www.dummies.com/extras/preventingreversingheartdisease.

In this part . . .

- ✔ Explore the basic lifestyle modifications you can make and the daily steps you can take to achieve heart health for you and your family.

- ✔ Follow guidelines and tips for creating a productive partnership with your doctor (or doctors).

- ✔ Discover the basics of good nutrition, a heart-healthy way of eating, and steps to incorporate adequate physical activity into your daily life.

- ✔ Foster good health by going beyond nutrition and exercise to tap into the mind/body connection.

- ✔ Learn strategies to achieve heart health and well-being for the whole family.

Chapter 4

Forming a Partnership with Your Doctor for the Best Heart Care

*I*n the words of comedienne Joan Rivers, "Can we talk?" Talking, of course, is exactly what you and your doctor need to do if you want to prevent heart disease. Throughout this book, one of my mantras is "forming a partnership with your physician."

Preventing heart disease starts with controlling risk factors. Even if you are the picture of perfect health — at least in the mirror — only regular checkups with your primary-care physician can tell you what's happening inside your body where many important coronary heart disease (CHD) risk factors silently get started. These include high blood pressure, cholesterol problems (dyslipidemia), and elevated blood sugar or insulin resistance. Even if you eat a heart-healthy diet, exercise regularly, and maintain an ideal weight, you need regular checkups. For a few people, inherited factors may increase risk of heart disease despite a healthy lifestyle. So think of your doctor as a valued consultant, who can confirm your good work or sound an early warning if early risks appear.

If you already have one or more risk factors for heart disease (most American adults have at least one), have been diagnosed with heart disease, or have experienced a heart attack or other event, then you must have good working relationships with all your physicians. Fighting so serious a foe as heart disease is not a battle to take on by yourself. You need the right heath-care team.

Finding the right physician and cardiologist, however, in the mazes of the medical system is not always easy. Neither is knowing how to establish clear lines of communication and cooperation. Hence, I've written this chapter. Think of it as a primer on partnership.

Building a Solid Healthcare Partnership

Like all partnerships — whether business relationships, marriages, or friendships — patient-physician partnerships must be based on open communication and trust. At its best, a partnership between you and your physician can be a long-term, trusting relationship with benefits to your cardiovascular and total health. Discussing how to optimize your cardio-vascular health with your physician also should be a pleasure to which you and your doctor look forward.

Many doctors, it pains me to say, are not willing, able, or ready to accept this kind of a partnership with their patients. But I believe that every patient needs to be a good consumer. That means you need to have realistic goals and realistically high expectations when selecting and working with a per-sonal physician and, if you need them, a cardiologist and other specialists.

Of course, your healthcare choices extend beyond finding the right physi-cians, so I offer tips for choosing a managed-care plan and a hospital, as well.

Selecting a primary-care doctor

Almost invariably, people, including those who have heart disease, depend upon their primary-care doctor for most of their healthcare needs. I've always been surprised by how randomly many people choose a physician. You need to regard your physician as a consultant in the same way you regard your accountant or your lawyer, and take the same care in choosing him or her.

First, look for a doctor who has superior knowledge about medicine, who listens, who asks pertinent questions, and who provides useful explanations and answers. Also look for a physician who displays genuine concern, cost-consciousness, and a determination to keep working on *any* medical problem that you have. Above all, your doctor needs to be someone who cares about you and inspires confidence, optimism, and hope in you.

A good way to begin identifying such candidates is by asking neighbors, family, or friends for recommendations. You can also obtain information or referrals by contacting local hospitals, medical schools, or medical societies. Many hospitals, clinics, and private practices now have websites where you likewise can obtain basic information. Profiles of individual physicians on these websites will usually enable you to get some basic information about the physician: where he or she went to medical school and trained after medi-cal school, focus areas of his or her practice, and research interests (if any). In addition, you may wish to look at local websites where current or former patients evaluate and score their doctor. Though such reviews are subjective, a doctor with high scores may deserve a further look.

Narrow down your choices to two or three physician candidates. Be sure that they are in your insurance network; you can determine this on your insurance plan's website. Then call their offices to arrange a time to speak with them, either in person or on the phone. This important preinterview enables you to find out how the physician approaches the world and his or her patients. Here are some questions you may want to ask during the preinterview:

- ✔ What are your special areas of medical interest?

- ✔ Can you tell me a little bit about how you approach medicine and patient care?

- ✔ In managing health and disease risk factors, how important to you are lifestyle factors, such as nutrition, physical activity and weight management?

- ✔ If you have an existing cardiac condition, ask these questions:

  - • What is your background in and knowledge of this particular condition?

  - • How do you typically manage heart disease risk factors? Do you focus on lifestyle measures first before using medications?

Be careful when asking these last questions, because even some of the very best physicians may be thrown off-guard by them, at least until they get to know you better.

When you're considering the answers to your questions and just how the conversation went in general, don't forget that who you are as an individual plays a role of utmost importance in deciding which doctor is best for you. Some people like detailed and thorough explanations. Others want a more regimented approach with less specific information. Don't be embarrassed to interview a few physicians to find out whether they fit best with who you are. Remember, you're establishing a long-term partnership here, so you should not rush into it.

Finding the right cardiologist

If you already have heart disease, you're going to be best cared for by both your family doctor and a cardiologist. A cardiologist has advanced training in *cardiology,* which is a subspecialty of internal medicine. Pursuing such a sub-specialty typically means anywhere from three to five years of training in addition to full training in internal medicine.

Choosing a cardiologist can be a little trickier than choosing a family care doctor, because the normal sources of information — family and friends — may not be as familiar with cardiology specialists, or you may belong to an insurance or managed-care plan that requires you to select from a particular group of physicians or to be referred by your primary-care physician. In fact, in most cases, your primary-care physician will refer you to a cardiologist. You can begin your search by asking your primary-care physician these questions about the cardiologists he or she recommends:

✔ Where did the cardiologist train?

✔ What are his or her areas of specialty within cardiology?

✔ At what hospitals does the cardiologist practice?

✔ How does the cardiologist approach his or her patients?

✔ Is the cardiologist willing to form partnerships and talk to patients, rather than merely giving directions and demanding that they be followed?

✔ How accessible is the cardiologist?

✔ How is the cardiologist as a human being?

On the basis of this information, you may treat your first consultation with the cardiologist as an opportunity to get better acquainted with his or her ideas and style. Use some of the same questions you would ask a primary-care physician. If you don't think the fit between the two of you is good, ask your primary-care physician for another referral. If you have found another candidate based on your research, ask your primary-care doctor for his or her opinion and a referral.

Choosing and working with a managed-care plan

In this day and age, the majority of Americans get their basic medical care through some form of managed-care plan, whether it's an HMO (health-maintenance organization), PPO (preferred-provider organization), or some other member of the Alphabet City of managed care.

If you receive your insurance through your employer, the way many Americans do, you may even be offered a choice of plans or choices within a single plan. If so, don't make the common mistake of basing your choice solely on cost. (That isn't how you chose your car, is it?) Instead, look carefully at these issues:

✔ Access to the physicians you want to see

✔ The qualifications of the physicians who have chosen the plan

✔ The hospitals that are affiliated with the plan

> ✔ Logistical issues such as convenience of doctors and hospitals to you
>
> ✔ If you have an established cardiac condition, the availability of certain treatments through the managed-care plan

Your human resources professional at work should be able to help you sort through these issues. Most managed-care plans have their own websites, so you can search the Internet for information on each plan.

If you must provide your own health insurance, you may have a more difficult time finding an affordable plan that gives you the coverage you want. Although the Affordable Care Act has made it possible for more people (such as those with pre-existing conditions) to get coverage, finding a plan that meets your needs can still take work. For example, many insurance plans have "narrow networks," with limited providers. Does the individual plan include your physicians and hospitals near you? Is a plan purchased through the government-sponsored Insurance Marketplace or is it one purchased directly from an insurance company right for your needs? Also check with insurance agents and with friends who are self-employed or purchase their insurance individually .

Hunting down a hospital

Choosing a hospital is a surprisingly important healthcare decision, particularly when you have cardiac disease. Recent studies show that patients at certain hospitals tend to have better outcomes. As a general rule, these hospitals are the ones that have programs for physicians in training. If your primary-care physician or cardiologist plans to refer you to a hospital for advanced testing or surgery, don't be shy about asking about the hospital's expertise and experience with these procedures. If I were facing open-heart surgery, for instance, I'd surely want to be in the care of a hospital team that specializes in that kind of surgery, performs it frequently (like every day!), and has an outstanding record of success and care. You can also now check out hospital ratings, based on reports hospitals have to do for the government and for accreditation and certification. Medicare's Hospital Compare (www.medicare.gov/hospitalcompare/search.html) and ratings by Consumer Reports (www.consumerreports.org) are both reliable.

If you already have established heart disease, I advise you to choose a large hospital with experience in cardiac care and a training program, if possible. Within medicine, these hospitals typically are *tertiary care hospitals,* which means they specialize in caring for patients with many advanced illnesses, including severe forms of heart disease. These hospitals usually can be identified through local medical societies or local or regional medical schools in your area.

Establishing a Partnership with Your Physician

Establishing an effective partnership between you and your physician requires four key elements.

✔ **Communication:** Open communication, the foundation of partnership, is clearly a two-way street.

- You have the right to expect your physician to fully and openly give you the information that helps you understand your condition and participate in your treatment.

- By the same token, your physician has the right to expect you to be frank about the symptoms you're experiencing, not only from your condition but also from any medicines you're taking. You should also tell your doctor about any over-the counter medications and supplements you take and any alternative therapies because these could affect your other medicines and symptoms.

✔ **Trust:** Trust enables both communication and commitment in partnership. You must trust that your physician always has your best interests at heart and that your physician is competent, caring, and concerned about your well-being. By the same token, your physician has to be able to trust that you're committed to your own well-being.

✔ **Commitment to the treatment plan:** Your responsibility within the partnership is to be committed to a treatment plan that you and your doctor agree upon. You shouldn't agree to a treatment plan unless you intend to carry it out.

You also need to be committed to finding out all that you can about your condition and the whys and wherefores of various treatment procedures. Ask again if you don't understand something. Ask your doctor for information. Use reputable print and online resources (such as the ones recommended throughout this book) to educate yourself. The more informed and knowledgeable you are, the more committed and equal a partner you're likely to be.

✔ **Quality care:** Your physician bears responsibility for quality care, not only as a function of his or her knowledge and integrity but also as a function of the total healthcare system serving you. Ensuring that any other physicians involved in your care also practice quality care is your physician's responsibility. All of the facilities associated with that system — including the office and the hospital and the performance of all the individuals within those settings — ultimately are the responsibility of the physician.

Communication and trust are elements shared between you and your doctor. Commitment to a treatment plan is your domain, and the quality of your care is your physician's.

Identifying what you have a right to expect of your physician

As a consumer, you have the right to expect that your physician will

- ✓ Listen carefully and provide thorough, clear explanations for procedures, conditions, and treatment options
- ✓ Answer your questions
- ✓ Possess the skills and knowledge of a physician committed to ongoing medical education and at the cutting edge of medical science

If your physician is not meeting these expectations, then it's time to look for another doctor.

Looking at what your physician has a right to expect of you

Yes, we docs have the right to some expectations, too. I can tell you, as a physician, nothing is more frustrating than trying to control blood pressure in people who intermittently take their medicine or trying to control blood lipids such as cholesterol in patients who don't pay attention to even the basics of sound nutrition and physical activity. You need to be your own best friend when it comes to your own medical care.

Your commitment is so important that I'm going to reemphasize these points:

- ✓ If you have reservations or doubts about the treatment plan your doctor proposes, discuss these problems fully with your physician before agreeing to the plan. Remember that you can always seek a second opinion from another doctor if the proposed treatment plan seems wrong to you.
- ✓ After you agree upon a plan, do it — and stick to it. If any problems, symptoms, or side effects arise, tell your doctor. Pick up the phone and tell the receptionist or nurse (whoever serves as the gatekeeper for incoming calls) exactly why you need to talk to the doctor.

✔ Be sure to follow the lifestyle measures. These are the foundation of your treatment. Preventing and possibly reversing heart disease is more than just taking a prescribed medication.

✔ Don't ever be ashamed to share your problems with your doctor. Nothing is shameful about having difficulties with making changes in your life. It is hard, but it is possible. You need the kind of relationship with your doctor that enables you to talk about your problems and not feel ashamed.

✔ Educate yourself about your condition.

Helping your primary-care doctor and cardiologist communicate

Although this topic may seem like a strange one to include, communication between your primary-care doctor and cardiologist is important. You're probably already thinking, "Shouldn't my doctors work with each other as a matter of course?" Naturally, they try their best to do that, but I can tell you that many times lab values and other critical information are lost, even in the best systems between the best doctors (even with the newest electronic records systems).

You can play an important role as a fail-safe communication link between your primary-care physician and your cardiologist. One way to accomplish this goal is making sure that the notes that go into your physician's record also are sent to you. Such notes include not only the impression of your progress from your primary-care doctor and your cardiologist but also any pertinent findings and laboratory values. Your medical record, by the way, is a legal document that belongs to you. It is an excellent idea to have your own portable health record file.

Optimizing office visits

Office visits to the doctor are a pain, aren't they? Particularly when you have to go out of town. So here are some tips for getting the most out of them.

✔ **Be efficient.** Respect your physician's time and expect that your physician will respect your time, too. If forms need to be completed, try to arrive a little early. Bring notes that track how you feel and any symptoms you're experiencing. If you've been referred by a primary-care physician, try to bring copies of pertinent medical records and lab tests. Bring a written list of the medications that you're taking, including the frequency and dosage. (Or you may wish to bring the actual medicines in their containers to the first visit.) If you have a discharge summary from a hospitalization, share it with your physician, particularly a sub-specialist such as a cardiologist. If you need to cancel your appointment, common courtesy mandates that you try to do so as early as possible. (The same goes for the physician.)

✔ **Describe your symptoms.** Be prepared to tell your doctor about any symptoms that you have, when they occur, how severe they are, and how they affect you. If it's a regular checkup and you have no complaints, be prepared to tell your doctor what you are doing to maintain good health (the diet you are eating, your level of physical activity, any weight loss or weight maintenance program you're on, and so on).

✔ **Bring notes.** Seeing your notes about the issues that you have always is beneficial to a physician, so write down your questions ahead of time. (That doesn't mean you can't also ask new ones as they arise.)

✔ **Ask about your diagnosis.** Asking specifically about your likely diagnosis and what tests the physician regards as important for specifically pinning down that diagnosis is important. Don't be afraid to ask for this information in layman's terms.

✔ **Take notes.** Many times, patients leave the doctor's office and forget what they discussed. Visiting the doctor is often stressful, so don't be afraid to take notes during the discussion and, for that matter, bring someone with you. A second pair of ears helps. Absent that, you can also record the conversation on your smartphone or tablet computer.

Whenever possible, ask for instructions in writing.

✔ **Schedule a follow-up appointment.** If a follow-up appointment is necessary, ask the doctor specifically when to schedule it. Asking how to reach the physician in case of an emergency also is important.

Tips for asking the right questions

Here are some recommended questions that you can ask your doctor about any condition that he or she may discover during an evaluation. You may even want to copy this list to take with you.

✔ What is my diagnosis?

✔ What tests will I need to undergo?

✔ Are there any side effects or dangers to these tests?

✔ What is the recommended treatment?

✔ What are the potential side effects of the treatment?

✔ Are there any treatment choices?

✔ Are there any other questions that I should be asking?

✔ Is there any source of information that I can read about my diagnosis?

Making testing easier

Most of us at some time face testing either to rule out a problem, confirm a diagnosis, or assess the efficacy of treatment. Wandering through a maze of unfamiliar hospital halls, chart and referral slip in hand, can be frightening and confusing. Avoid such anxiety and confusion by planning ahead.

✔ Ask your primary-care physician or your cardiologist exactly what tests you'll be undergoing and what the potential benefit and outcome of each of the tests or procedures will be.

✔ Ask for a map and/or directions to the testing center or hospital. If your physician's office doesn't have this information, check the testing center's website or call them for directions and be sure to find out where to park and where to check in.

✔ If they don't tell you up front, ask the technicians at each testing or procedure area exactly what will happen during the test, any side effects that you may feel, and what information the test is likely to reveal. Most technicians and physicians are delighted to explain their procedures.

Considering Special Issues in the Doctor-Patient Relationship

I've outlined some general rules for working with your physician. However, a few special circumstances may come up that you need to consider. The following sections look at a few of them.

Participating in research studies

Many physicians today are involved in clinical research. Most participate in these studies to further their knowledge and to keep up with modern medical advances. For the most part, clinical research is a good thing. Unfortunately, a few unscrupulous physicians engage in clinical research for monetary gain and sometimes pressure patients to enter research projects that may not be of benefit to them.

If your physician recommends that you enter a clinical research trial, you have the right to ask whether the therapy being studied has any recognized benefits. You also have the right to have a thorough explanation of why this therapy is being recommended and how it differs from regular therapy. Although I support clinical research, I think it is important that patients not be coerced (even subtly) into participating in clinical research trials — particularly when up-to-date therapies are established in almost every aspect of cardiovascular disease.

Getting your physician's attention when it's difficult

Nothing is more frustrating than having your physician ignore you when you have questions, concerns, or troubling symptoms. Unfortunately, many physician's offices screen calls in such a way that it's difficult to get through to the physician. Often an assistant, such as a nurse, takes your question, confers with the doctor, and calls you back. If you feel your concerns have been handled appropriately by this "physician extender," that's okay. If not, specifically request that the physician call you back to address your concern. If the physician is unwilling to do so after several phone calls, then write the physician a letter saying that you're concerned about his or her failure to call you back in a timely manner. If the doctor also ignores the written request, then it's time to look for a new physician. After all, would you accept that kind of treatment from your lawyer or accountant?

Getting a second opinion

You have a right to obtain a second opinion about any serious diagnosis. Second opinions are deeply respected in medicine. A good physician will never be offended if you seek a second opinion. After all, in many instances, two heads are better than one. Don't be embarrassed to ask your physician to recommend someone to offer a second opinion. If your physician is the kind of doctor that you want to see, he or she will have no problem with this straightforward request.

Changing to a new doctor when necessary

Switching physicians also is completely within your rights as a patient. Different patient and physician styles often do not mesh perfectly, which can hinder your ability to communicate adequately. You also need to trust that your physician has superior medical skills and knowledge. If you don't feel confident in either of these areas, it's time to start looking for another physician.

One word of caution: As you're considering the need to change, examine your own thinking and emotions for signs of denial. Sometimes when a physician gives a diagnosis that is difficult to accept, a patient may have the inclination to start looking around for a doctor who will offer a more comfortable, if less truthful, diagnosis. All too often, such "doctor shopping" leads to inferior care.

Chapter 5

Embracing a Healthy Diet and Active Lifestyle

In This Chapter

▶ Eating right while eating well

▶ Adopting simple nutrition principles for heart health and overall health

▶ Understanding why physical activity is important to heart health

▶ Planning your own physical activity program

*W*hat's the secret to keeping your heart healthy for life? Even if you already have risks for and/or manifestations of heart disease? Given the facts on heart disease I present in the previous two chapters, you may expect a complex response to these questions. But the basics for achieving heart health are really simple: Eat a heart-healthy diet and stay physically active. These two lifestyle practices are the foundation for heart health and overall health. Achieving both is easier and more fun than you might think. This chapter outlines simple, but proven, strategies you can adapt to your needs and goals.

Making Nutrition Work for You

As far as your heart goes, you are what you eat. Sound nutrition is critically important in maintaining and fostering heart health. The word *nutrition* grows out of an ancient Latin word meaning "to nourish" or "to suckle." How splendidly the root meaning of this word illustrates what eating well and eating right is all about, because mother's milk is a perfect blend of just the right amount of the nutrients that babies need for a good start. Likewise, good nutrition for all your days means good eating from the balanced variety of foods needed to support life and health.

In spite of all the food and diet hype that you hear, the guidelines for healthy eating I share in this chapter are simple and can withstand the tests of experience and science. Adopting them as the foundation of your enjoyment of food points you toward a healthy heart and optimal health. So don't let the word *nutrition* scare you; just think good eating for good health.

Whatever trouble people eat themselves into, they generally can eat themselves out of! Even though poor food choices, such as eating too many foods high in saturated fat or highly refined carbs, contribute to significant health problems, including heart disease, adopting some simple, commonsense approaches to modifying your food choices for the better can lower your risk of heart disease and help you manage almost all heart conditions. These same smart choices also can help you control weight problems (see Chapter 10) and improve health, happiness, and quality of life. Adding regular physical activity supports these dietary strategies. These choices won't, however, bring back a good ten-cent cup of coffee or improve the return on your IRA. You can't have everything.

Choosing Healthy Pleasures: Guidelines for Eating Right While Eating Well

Here's the first rule of heart-healthy eating: You can eat well in ways that improve your cardiac health without being a food cop.

Many people suffer from the misconception that healthy cooking takes all the pleasure out of eating by making food taste bland and unappetizing. No way! In fact, many of the top chefs in America now are creating recipes that not only are healthy but also are a pleasure to consume. Many home chefs are pretty expert, too — so why not you? Supporting you in this effort, I share heart-healthy recipes for each meal of the day in Part IV. You can find a many more in *The Healthy Heart Cookbook For Dummies,* written by yours truly, and *Mediterranean Diet Cookbook for Dummies,* by Meri Raffetto and Wendy Jo Peterson — both of which are published by John Wiley & Sons, Inc.

Eat a variety of nutritious whole foods daily

A number of major health and nutrition organizations in the U.S., including the Dietary Guidelines for Americans, the American Heart Association (AHA), and the Academy of Nutrition and Dietetics (formerly the American Dietetic Association), have developed basic principles for healthy nutrition. They continue to refine these principles as new research adds to the literally thousands of scientific studies upon which they're based. In this section I present the essential nutritional goals to remember in simple, commonsense statements.

Choose a variety of fruits and vegetables daily — at least five servings

Fruits and vegetables are important for what they do and do not contain. Fruits and vegetables are loaded with fiber, antioxidants, and other phytochemicals that lower the risks of heart disease and cancer. In addition, they are low in sodium, and most have no fat. As a result, fruits and vegetables don't increase blood pressure or blood cholesterol. Studies also show that people with high blood pressure who consume a diet containing high levels of fruits and vegetables and low-fat dairy products significantly reduced their blood pressure. Last, but hardly least, fruits and vegetables are a major source of the complex carbohydrates that are the body's primary source of fuel.

Extensive research confirms that eating a minimum of five servings of fruits and vegetables daily provides significant benefits to heart health and overall health. Eating more is also good, but the baseline you want to reach is five servings.

Select a variety of whole-grain foods daily

Whole-grain foods, such as whole-grain cereals, bread, pasta and brown rice, form a mainstay of heart-healthy eating along with fruits and vegetables, because they are very high in fiber and in complex carbohydrates. In addition to popular whole grains such as oats, wheat, rye, brown rice, and corn, other less familiar whole grains you might try include quinoa, barley, buckwheat, and amaranth.

Not consuming enough fiber clearly is associated with increased risk of heart disease. Everyone should be consuming approximately 25 grams of fiber from natural dietary sources every day, yet the sad truth is that most people eat only about half of this amount.

If you pay attention to popular media, you may get the impression that carbohydrates are the last thing you should eat. Actually, as I just noted, carbohydrates are the body's main source of energy. Has carbohydrate consumption contributed to the increased incidence of obesity in the U.S. as some claim? I would suggest that this assertion is misleading. Overconsumption of calories, coupled with inadequate physical activity, has led to the explosion of obesity in the U.S. Unfortunately, many of those extra calories have come from refined simple carbohydrates and added sugars, which essentially are *empty calories,* or calories that don't provide the nutritional punch of whole-grain foods and fruits and vegetables. So think and choose *whole grains!*

Choose lean protein foods

Protein provides the building blocks for the body's cells. Protein helps repair cells and build new ones and supports development for growing children and teens. Most Americans get enough protein and more. The goal is to select the most healthful proteins. If you eat animal protein, select lean cuts of meat and trim visible fat or remove poultry skin before or after cooking. Fish and nonfat or low-fat dairy and eggs also provide protein. You can also get adequate protein from plant sources such as dried beans, tofu and other soy foods, nuts and nut butters, seeds, some whole grains, and nondairy milks (such as soy and nut milks).

Getting protein aplenty

The average American eats much more protein than necessary — or optimal — for good health. Most of this protein is consumed in the form of meat. Although eating a high-protein diet can help with short-term weight loss, you may end up paying a significant price. High-protein diets usually are also high in fat and may increase cholesterol. Consuming an adequate amount of protein doesn't take much effort:

✔ Eating two 2- to 3-ounce servings of fish, lean meat, or poultry provides an adequate daily protein intake.

✔ Eating one egg or two egg whites provides protein equal to one ounce of meat or fish.

✔ Enjoying smaller portions of meat in combination main dishes such as pasta, stir-fries, or casseroles cuts back on protein consumption — just remember to avoid high fat.

✔ Adding tofu (soybean curd) to stir-fries and casseroles provides good protein with relatively low fat.

✔ Choosing bean dishes, particularly combos such as beans and rice, or beans and whole-grain pasta, gives you a good source of protein and fiber.

Enjoy healthy oils and fats in moderation

Just as it needs carbohydrates and protein, your body needs the right fats in the right amounts for good general health and good heart health. There are three types of healthful fats — monounsaturated fats (MUFAS), polyunsaturated fats (PUFAS), and omega-3 fatty acids:

✔ **Monounsaturated fats (MUFAS)** come from vegetable sources, such as olive, canola, and peanut oils, and foods such as nuts, seeds, olives, and avocados. Monounsaturated oils are typically liquid at room temperature. Substantial evidence suggests that monounsaturated fats, particularly the ways they are consumed in a Mediterranean diet that features olive oil, can significantly lower your risk of heart disease by helping to improve blood cholesterol (lipid) levels and fighting inflammation. They may also help control blood glucose levels, which helps control type 2 diabetes, a risk factor for heart disease. See the sidebar, "Checking out two heart-healthy diets" for information on Mediterranean diets.

✔ **Polyunsaturated fats (PUFAS)** also come primarily from vegetable sources and typically are liquid at room temperature. Corn oil and most other salad oils are examples of polyunsaturated oils. Polyunsaturated fats also help improve blood lipid levels and benefit control of type 2 diabetes.

✔ **Omega-3 fatty acids** are found in certain fatty fish, such as salmon, sardines, herring, lake trout, and canned light tuna (lower mercury than albacore tuna), as well as such plant foods as walnuts, flax seed, and canola and soybean oils. There is substantial evidence that omega 3s benefit heart health and help reduce heart disease risk. The American Heart Association recommends eating fish twice weekly (3.5-ounce cooked servings), except for pregnant women and children. Wild caught fish (sustainably fished) appear to have higher levels of mercury than farmed fish. Because of their high mercury content, avoid swordfish, king mackerel, tile fish, and shark; for current and local fish advisories, go to one of the webpages listed next, or enter "EPA Fish Consumption Advisories" in your Internet browser:

- **Advisories Where You Live Map** (`http://fishadvisoryonline.epa.gov/General.aspx`): Simply enter in a body of water on the map to see advisories in your area.

- **Fish Consumption Advisory** (`http://water.epa.gov/scitech/swguidance/fishshellfish/fishadvisories/`): This site provides a one-stop shop, including links to general advisories/info, as well as a link to the Advisories Where You Live Map.

Although these oils and fats can contribute to good nutrition and heart health, they have a potential downside: Like all fats, they are high calorie. At nine calories per gram, they have more than twice the four calories per gram of carbohydrates and protein. Eating too many foods high in fat contributes to the overconsumption of calories by most Americans. So what's the best policy? Substitute healthful fats for saturated fats; don't simply increase the amount you eat.

What's the story on dietary supplements?

Since many observational studies report positive links to the intake of certain vitamins, minerals, and antioxidants with better heart health, you might think that taking supplements offers good insurance for heart health. However, a number of recent randomized clinical trials have not confirmed that link and have offered mixed results.

The first, and best, way to get the vitamins, minerals, antioxidants, and other nutrients your body needs is to eat a balanced diet that contains a variety of whole foods. Research suggests that the complex mix of nutrients and dietary factors founds in fruits, vegetables, whole grains, and other whole foods work together in beneficial ways that aren't matched by taking a single substance.

If you have heart disease, you physician may recommend taking an omega-3 supplement. However, many common supplements, particularly herbals, may interact in potentially dangerous ways with various heart medications. Be sure to discuss any supplements you are thinking of taking with your physician.

The best advice for fostering heart health and general health and preventing chronic disease is to eat a balanced diet of healthy foods. If you feel that your diet may be deficient in any area, again discuss it with your doctor before taking any supplement. If you choose to take supplements, don't exceed the daily recommended levels.

Limit sodium, problem fats, and energy-dense foods

Another aspect of heart-healthy nutrition is making food choices that limit intakes of certain ingredients that can work against heart health. The most important things to limit are sodium (salt), saturated fats and trans fats, and energy-dense foods that provide energy (calories) but relatively few nutrients.

Use less salt and choose prepared foods with less salt

Guidelines currently recommend that adults in general should consume less than 2,300 milligrams of sodium daily, about 1 teaspoon of table salt (sodium chloride). The recommendation is less than 1,500 milligrams daily (just over a half teaspoon salt) for adults 51 and older, individuals of African American heritage, and anyone with high blood pressure, diabetes, or a diagnosis of heart disease. On average, most American adults consume about twice the recommended amount. Now, I know you don't sprinkle that much salt over your food at the table, but many prepared and convenience foods have high levels of sodium — take a glance at the labels. The same goes for restaurant offerings, whether they're fast food or haute cuisine.

The major reason to limit salt/sodium intake has to do with its association with high blood pressure. In societies where less sodium is consumed, the incidence of high blood pressure is dramatically lower than it is in the U.S. If people with hypertension pay more attention to strict limitations on salt consumption and control their weight, many can manage blood pressure without medications.

Consume fewer foods with saturated fats and avoid trans fats

Eating too much saturated fat, especially trans fat, contributes to elevated total cholesterol and LDL cholesterol (the bad kind), which have clear links to developing atherosclerosis, including that of coronary heart disease. Saturated fat also is linked to diabetes and colon cancer. Here's what you need to know:

- **Saturated fats (SFA)** typically come from animal sources, such as fat in meat and poultry and butterfat in dairy products; some fats from tropical plants, such as cocoa butter, palm oil, and coconut oil, also are saturated. Saturated fats typically are solid at room temperature. Good ways to lower your intake of saturated fats are to substitute healthy fats, trim all visible fat from meat, and eat nonfat or low-fat dairy products.

- **Trans fat** is a saturated fat that is made by adding hydrogen to vegetable oil, turning it into a solid. Hydrogenation makes the oil stable and helps prevent it from going rancid; that's why trans fats are used in many manufactured foods. Vegetable shortening and stick margarine are two examples of trans fats. Trans fat, which is labeled as *hydrogenated* or *partially hydrogenated vegetable oil,* raises unhealthy LDL cholesterol and may lower healthy HDL cholesterol. Avoid trans fat entirely if possible.

From a dietary point of view, the first line of therapy for elevated cholesterol is lowering your intake of saturated fats and trans fats. Although dietary cholesterol is not as big an influence on blood cholesterol as saturated fat and trans fat, limiting the amount of cholesterol you eat is still important, particularly if you have diabetes. Cholesterol is found in animal foods. The recommended daily intake level is 300 milligrams. To put this in perspective, note that the yolk of an average egg contains 215 mg of cholesterol. Egg whites, on the other hand, are cholesterol-free.

Adding healthy zip to your food

Cutting fat, cholesterol, and salt doesn't necessarily mean cutting flavor. Keeping these five items on hand gives me plenty of ways to add some zip to food, while eating a low-fat and low-salt diet.

- ✔ **Vegetable and fruit salsas:** From party dips to dressings for salads or vegetables to sauces for fish, salsas are versatile. Find a good prepared salsa to keep on hand (watch out for too much sodium) and experiment with your own freshly made combinations.

- ✔ **Chilis:** Some like it hot! Supermarkets these days offer a good range of peppers hot and hotter. And for the pantry shelf, hundreds of hot sauces are available. You use so little that sodium usually isn't a problem. From the Caribbean to Asia and the entire globe in between, every style of cooking has creative uses for the pepper. It's a kick that won't hurt you.

- ✔ **Mustards:** Did you know hundreds of different mustards are on the market, ready for you to use? Mustards are a great substitute for traditional fats in dressing everything from sandwiches to entrees. Some can be pretty high in sodium (salt), but a little mustard goes a long way.

- ✔ **Balsamic (and other) vinegars:** A good balsamic vinegar is so nutty and sweet that many folks enjoy it alone as a salad dressing or on a sandwich. Try the many specialty and flavored vinegars available to add a piquant touch to much more than just salads.

- ✔ **Fresh (or dried) herbs:** Dill, basil, cilantro, thyme, rosemary, oregano, chives . . . just the names make my mouth water. Supermarkets now carry a wider range of fresh herbs, and during growing season, you'll find lots at farmers' markets or you can grow them yourself. After you taste what fresh basil can do for a tomato or pasta or what a rosemary sprig and lemon juice can do for a grilled fish filet or chicken breast, you'll be looking for more opportunities to use fresh herbs.

Look Mom, low cholesterol!

Dietary cholesterol, which is found exclusively in animal tissue, is more prevalent in eggs and organ meats. Here some tips for avoiding it.

Eggs: Most people know that eggs are high in cholesterol. One average egg yolk has 215 mg. But you can have your eggs and avoid cholesterol, too.

✔ Substitute two egg whites (0 mg cholesterol) for one whole egg in almost any recipe in which the egg doesn't star.

✔ Use egg substitute or cholesterol-free egg products.

✔ For scrambled eggs and omelets, use one whole egg and one egg white instead of two whole eggs.

Organ meats: Liver, for instance, is just loaded with cholesterol. One 3-ounce slice of beef liver has 410 mg; one chicken liver has 125 mg. So if you like organ meats, save brains, sweetbreads, gizzards, hearts, and kidneys for a treat. If you hate liver, here's an excuse never to eat it again.

Choose foods to moderate your intake of energy-dense foods

Who doesn't like a little something sweet or a savory snack? Unfortunately, most Americans consume far too many empty calories in the form of cookies, ice cream, candy, soft drinks and other sweet treats or savory snacks. We also like foods and snacks made out of highly refined flours, which don't have the fiber and nutrients of whole grains. (The intake of highly refined carbohydrates has also been linked to increased levels of small dense LDL cholesterol.)

So think about these possible choices: One average candy bar or one half-cup serving of a premium ice cream contains about 275 to 300 calories (much of which is sugar and fat). For the same number of calories, you can eat two to three bananas, pears, or apples; or three to four peaches, apricots, or plums; an entire cantaloupe; a big wedge of watermelon; or a quart-and-a-half of strawberries. Or you could eat a whole bowl of air-popped or microwaved low-fat, whole-grain popcorn. You no doubt get my drift. Plenty of good-for-you treats are available. Go ahead and enjoy the occasional ice cream, candy, or soda, but for everyday eating, think in terms of "more is less" — more fruit (more nutrition) is less caloric intake.

If you consume alcohol, do so in moderation

From a cardiovascular point of view, alcohol consumption is a complex issue. Moderate alcohol consumption actually has been shown to lower the risk of heart attack. Yet alcohol also is loaded with calories and may, therefore, contribute to weight gain. Furthermore, excessive alcohol consumption actually carries with it the cardiovascular risk of increasing blood pressure and acting in adverse ways on the cardiac muscle itself.

Research and debate continue about the complex mechanisms (including genetic links) and pathways through which alcohol appears to benefit heart health. Debate also continues about which type of alcohol (wine, beer, spirits) may hold the advantage, although red wine in particular has received a lot of study.

Moderate alcohol consumption generally is defined as no more than one drink daily for women and two drinks for men. One drink equals a 1.5 shot of distilled spirits, 5 ounces of wine, or 12 ounces of beer. Higher levels of alcohol consumption carry unacceptable health risks.

Balance the energy you eat with the energy you burn

Obesity is a major risk factor for a variety of health consequences, but particularly for heart disease. About 75 percent of all mortality associated with obesity comes from the increased risk of heart disease. Regular physical activity burns more calories, helps raise your metabolism, helps you maintain lean muscle, and helps keep your heart strong and healthy. Most Americans enjoy eating, and, if you are physically active, you can consume a few more calories than if you are sedentary — just remember to make your choices nutrient dense.

How much should you eat to maintain your weight? Check out Chapter 10 for a daily calorie guide that takes into account age and activity level. For a BMI calculator and BMI tables, go to `http://www.nhlbi.nih.gov/health/educational/lose_wt/BMI/bmicalc.htm` to see where your current weight falls — underweight, normal, overweight, obese.

Counting ketchup as a vegetable? Tips for heart-healthy dining out

Eat at some fast food eateries on a regular basis, and you'd certainly have to count ketchup as a vegetable to have any hope of eating your daily five. And don't even think about avoiding excess fat! But dining out need not be so fraught with peril for your healthy eating goals. If you keep these simple tips in mind, you can eat out, eat well, and eat right:

✔ **Select a restaurant that can help you stay on plan.** Whether you're headed out for fine dining or fast food (or anything in between), you can choose a restaurant that helps you meet your goals. For example, a sandwich shop where you can select lean ingredients and toppings may be a better choice than a place that offers only burgers and fries. The same sort of distinctions also can apply at better restaurants.

✔ **Order wisely to make the menu work for you.** Almost every restaurant offers items and/or methods of preparation that you can enjoy with a cheerful heart. Make the menu work for you with wise selections:

- Broiled, baked, or roasted rather than fried

- Vegetable or clear sauces rather than butter or cream sauces

- Steamed rather than creamed or fried veggies

- Dressing on the side for your salad

✔ **Practice portion control.** "Bigger is better" seems to be the catchphrase for portions at many restaurants. When presented with a plate heaped with enough for two or three, resist temptation — eat what you need, and take the rest home to Fido, or leave it. Where available, use calorie information to inform your choices. If the restaurant deserves a repeat visit, maybe you can share that great dish with a friend. You can also order an appetizer as an entree or seek restaurants that specialize in small-plate offerings.

✔ **Enjoy the occasional blowout.** Remember that Greek tyrant Procrustes who chopped off chunks of visitors to fit his guest bed? That isn't what heart-healthy eating is about. If a juicy steak with all the trimmings or a classic French dinner with great wine is your idea of the proper way to celebrate, *bon appetit!* Healthy eating is about overall moderation and balance. Only one caution: If your cardiologist has told you to avoid certain practices, pay close attention.

Checking out two heart-healthy diets

For a long time, doctors and dietitians have known that residents of the countries around the Mediterranean Sea seem to have a lower incidence of heart disease than is the case in most other countries. Many argue that the so-called Mediterranean diet, which is high in monounsaturated fats (largely from olive oil), grains, and vegetables, makes a major contribution to the low incidence of heart disease in this region. Monounsaturated fats seem to raise the HDL (the good cholesterol) but not total cholesterol. The American Heart Association and the Academy of Nutrition and Dietetics have increasingly used Mediterranean-styled diets as recommendations for lowering your risk of chronic disease. One downside of any oil, however, is that it's loaded with calories. Just remember to use oil in moderation.

Although the *DASH Diet* was designed as part of a research study that tested the effect of dietary patterns on preventing and lowering high blood pressure, it offers an excellent approach for general heart health. DASH stands for *Dietary Approaches to Stop Hypertension,* an eating plan that reduces total and saturated fat intake and emphasizes fruits, vegetables, and low-fat dairy foods. It also limits your intake of sweets. Read all about the DASH Diet on the DASH page (http://www.nhlbi.nih.gov/health/resources/heart/hbp-dash-index.htm) of the website of the National Heart, Lung, and Blood Institute (NHLBI), the study's sponsor.

Understanding Physical Activity and What It Can Do for Heart Health

The good news is that physical activity not only helps prevent heart disease, but it also plays an important role in the therapy for people who have various cardiac conditions. The principles that I discuss in this section are appropriate for both situations, but I want to emphasize clearly that if you have existing heart disease, you must carefully discuss physical activity with your personal physician so that together you can plan an activity program that's appropriate for you and your particular condition. With that caution in mind, physical activity offers many health benefits for everyone.

Recognizing the difference between physical activity and exercise

Once when I was giving a speech about the importance of regular physical activity for heart health, a woman stood up and said, "That may be important, but I had my fill of wearing gym shorts back in grade school. I'll never do it again!"

This woman was expressing the classic confusion between exercise and physical activity. Although considerable overlap exists between the two, they are not exactly the same:

- ✔ **Physical activity** is a much broader concept than exercise and can be defined as any muscular movement that utilizes energy. Sitting on your couch, for example, is not physical activity. Getting your butt off of that couch is!

- ✔ **Exercise** is a *type* of physical activity that typically is defined more narrowly as a planned and structured activity where bodily movements are repeated to achieve various aspects of fitness. Most people usually think of exercise as activities such as aerobic dance, running, swimming laps, or resistance training with weights.

 Drawing a distinction between physical activity and exercise may seem like nit-picking, but the distinction is important from a practical standpoint. Many people don't realize that simply getting out of their easy chairs and raking the leaves on a brisk autumn day or spending an hour gardening classifies as physical activity and that such physical activity during a lifetime has been shown to lower the risk of heart disease.

Identifying the benefits of physical activity

Regular physical activity fosters good health and helps prevent heart disease and other chronic conditions such as obesity, high blood pressure, cancer, and diabetes. Here I outline some of the specific benefits physical activity offers for your heart health.

Fostering primary prevention of heart disease

Even if you feel fine and fit and have no risk factors for heart disease, you can experience several positive changes after just two or three months of regular physical activity:

✓ Tasks that previously made you short of breath are easier to perform.

✓ Your heart rate when you're resting is lower. Because a more efficient heart pumps more blood on each beat, it requires fewer beats per minute to supply your body with oxygen when you're simply sitting still.

✓ Your heart is a stronger muscle. During a lifetime of moderate physical activity, the heart, as a muscle, maintains better condition than the heart of someone who remains or becomes inactive.

✓ The coronary arteries, which supply blood to the heart, are more likely to stay large and relatively clean in individuals who exercise on a regular basis. Remember that clean coronary arteries prevent heart attacks (see Chapter 2).

Reducing risk factors for heart disease

Regular physical activity can help you reduce many risk factors for heart disease. Reducing risks makes it much less likely that you will develop heart disease. Regular activity helps you do the following:

✓ **Manage high blood pressure (hypertension):** Regular physical activity not only reduces the risk of developing hypertension, but it also is an effective treatment for hypertension. (See Chapter 8 for details.)

✓ **Improve unhealthy cholesterol levels:** Physical activity can help raise HDL cholesterol and may help lower LDL cholesterol, particularly in people who have been inactive and have poor diets when they begin. Physical activity also appears to help increase the size of lipoproteins carrying cholesterol; larger particles are not as dangerous as small, dense LDL particles.

✔ **Prevent diabetes:** Physical activity also is a great way of lowering your risk of diabetes. Studies show that physically active people reduce their risks of adult onset diabetes between 24 percent and 100 percent.

✔ **Achieve and maintain a healthy body weight:** People who are inactive are much more likely to gain weight during their lives than people who are physically active. The expenditure of calories on a regular basis also tends to preserve lean muscle mass and make you capable of increased levels of functioning throughout your life.

✔ **Improve mental and emotional states:** Numerous studies show that physical activity reduces anxiety and tension and can improve mood and decrease the likelihood of depression.

✔ **Maintain functional fitness as you get older.** Physical activity has been shown to benefit older adults, too. If you reach the age of 65, you have an 80 percent chance of reaching the age of 80! Reducing your risk of heart disease and contributing risk factors such as high cholesterol, high blood pressure, and diabetes, and keeping the heart and muscles in tune and able to perform activities of daily living is particularly important for older individuals.

Benefiting secondary prevention of heart disease

Even if you have been diagnosed with atherosclerosis or had cardiac symptoms or a heart event, physical activity is an important part of your treatment regimen. It helps you do the following:

✔ **Reduce the risks of coronary heart disease (CHD):** Physical activity programs can help people who experience angina or who have been diagnosed with CHD increase their ability to perform activities of daily life and lower their risk of having additional problems.

✔ **Reduce the risk of another heart attack or heart event:** If you've suffered a heart attack, a supervised cardiac rehabilitation program under the guidance of a trained cardiologist (see Chapter 15) can help strengthen your damaged heart and help it function more efficiently. A fit body requires less work from the heart. Physical activity also helps prevent a second heart event by helping you reduce risk factors.

✔ **Increasing the efficiency of your muscles so they require less blood flow from the heart:** In the normal heart, approximately 70 percent to 80 percent of the blood that is returned to the heart is pumped out with each beat. After a heart attack or in the case of heart failure, the heart may pump much less blood out with each beat. Appropriate lower-intensity physical activity can help you to increase the efficiency of your muscles so that they make lower demands on the heart.

Understanding How Much Physical Activity Is Enough

How much physical activity do you need to promote good heart health and reduce the risks of heart disease? To start, let me say that *any* amount of activity is better than *none*! However, extensive research has determined the following levels of activity at which you can achieve many of the benefits of physical activity for heart health and overall health:

- ✔ **Adults:** Adults should achieve the following activity levels:
  - At least 150 minutes weekly of moderate intensity activity, or,
  - At least 75 minutes weekly of vigorous intensity activity, or,
  - A combination of both

  Increasing to 300 minutes weekly of moderate activity or 150 minutes of vigorous activity (or a combo) provides even more benefits.

- ✔ **Children:** Children need 60 minutes daily of moderate to vigorous intensity activity.

These findings are reflected in the recommendations of the Physical Activity Guidelines for Americans, the American Heart Association, American College of Sports Medicine, and other authoritative bodies.

The most beneficial pattern for most people is probably to get 30 minutes of activity on five days of the week. But here's a surprise — you need not exercise in one 30-minute bout. Accumulating three 10-minute bouts in a day is also effective. Guidelines also recommend adding two days of resistance training to help strengthen muscles and maintain muscle mass.

Judging moderate intensity

Moderate intensity activities provide a level of exertion that is between light and heavy. In other words, the type of activity that you choose needs to be intense enough so that you know you're exerting yourself, but not so intense that you're out of breath with sweat pouring.

Examples of moderate activity include brisk walking, slow swimming, leisurely cycling, mowing the lawn, raking the yard, and vacuuming.

If you charge into exercise, you'll wear yourself out at best and injure yourself at worst (particularly if you have a heart problem). Here are four basic ways to make sure that you stay within the *moderate* exertion zone.

- **Take the talk test.** Make sure that you can carry on a normal conversation with a companion while you're engaged in a bout of physical activity.

- **Check out your perceived exertion.** Pay attention to your body. Ask yourself, "Am I exerting myself at a moderate level, or am I actually exerting myself at a light level or heavy level?" Be honest with yourself. (Nobody but you is going to blab.) Research shows that by using this subjective gauge, most people can accurately determine whether they're working at a moderate intensity level of exertion.

If you have high blood pressure, talk to your doctor about appropriate intensity levels. Individuals with high blood pressure or angina, for instance, usually need to work at light-moderate or lower-intensity levels.

- **Take your pulse.** With a little practice, you can find your pulse on the thumb side of the inside of the wrist. Count your pulse for ten seconds and then multiply by six to find out your heart rate in beats per minute during exertion. Moderate exertion for a healthy individual takes place between 60 and 70 percent of your predicted maximum heart rate. For individuals with high blood pressure or a heart condition, moderate exertion takes place at lower percentages of maximum exertion, so ask your physician for specific instructions.

To estimate your maximum heart rate, subtract your age in years from 220 beats per minute. Thus, for a 40-year-old individual, the predicted maximum heart rate is 220 beats minus 40 beats — 180 beats per minute. The moderate exertion level of 60 percent to 70 percent of 180 beats equals 108 to 126 beats per minute.

- **Use a heart-rate monitor.** You can find inexpensive heart-rate monitors on the market that accurately keep track of your heartbeat during exercise and take the hassle out of accurately determining your exertion level. I particularly recommend the use of a heart-rate monitor if you have high blood pressure or any type of heart disease, or if you've experienced a heart attack.

Thinking no pain, no gain? No way!

Many people mistakenly think that exercise needs to be painful to be beneficial. Nothing could be farther from the truth, particularly when you have heart disease. In fact, if exercise is painful, it probably isn't good for anyone. Furthermore, for heart patients, pain, particularly chest pain, typically is a warning sign that you're exerting yourself too hard. Slow down.

Choosing the Right Activity for You

People often ask me what is the best activity or exercise to promote heart health and general fitness. My answer never changes: It is the form of exercise that you will do! Look at *all* the things you like to do, because somewhere in that list is an activity that will get you started. Also ask yourself what is convenient? What have I done successfully in the past? And then answer the questions honestly. (No daydreams of making the next Olympic team.)

For many people, the answer to these questions is walking. For others (depending on heart health, too), the physical activity of choice may be swimming, running, tai chi, aerobic dance, zumba, yoga, in-line skating, or other forms of regular exertion.

Avoid the deadly home-gym syndrome. Don't get me wrong . . . I'm not against fitness equipment. In fact, I have three or four pieces of home fitness equipment in my workout area. But be realistic and choose forms of exercise that are simple, enjoyable, and convenient. Too many of my patients and friends have expensive clothes racks, so make sure you enjoy using such equipment before you purchase it. A month's no-contract gym membership may help you decide.

Planning your activity program

Don't make your program too complex. I suggest that you start with a simple aerobic activity — I highly recommend walking — and build up your program from there.

Start your program with aerobic exercise

Every beginning exerciser needs to build his or her program around a core of what are called *aerobic* exercises. *Aerobic* literally means "in the presence of air." So aerobic exercises are those that require your muscles to burn more oxygen and you to breathe faster. Hard-working, air-hungry muscles demand more oxygen-rich blood from the heart. The heart in turn works a little harder and grows stronger. In this way, aerobic exercise helps lower the risk of heart disease. Although you work at lower levels of intensity when you already have heart disease, aerobic activity still will be the foundation of your activity program.

You can mix and match activities. Many different kinds of aerobic activities and exercises exist. All of them are good for the heart. Pick the ones that you think may be most convenient for you, or, better yet, mix and match. I also need to emphasize that daily forms of physical activity, such as leaf raking, lawn work, gardening, even brisk housework, all qualify as *moderate* physical activity and all are equally beneficial for the heart. Make them part of your overall plan.

Here are some aerobic activities you might enjoy:

- Walking
- Aerobic dance
- Cross-country skiing
- Cycling, outdoors
- Cycling, stationary
- Dancing, jazz, modern, tap

- In-line skating
- Rowing
- Running/jogging
- Stair climbing
- Swimming
- Zumba

Involve your physician

Preventing or managing heart disease requires teamwork. As I said earlier, let your doctor know of your desire to participate in a program of regular physical activity and seek his or her guidance. Your doctor can help you fine-tune your physical activity program to account for your unique personal circumstances such as current medications, current level of physical activity, and current physical conditions, including existing heart disease. You may consider having an exercise tolerance test before starting to exercise.

If you already have any heart condition, taking an exercise tolerance test prior to starting a program of physical activity is important. Guidelines indicate that men older than the age of 50 and women older than the age of 55 who've lived previously sedentary lifestyles should also have a physician-supervised exercise tolerance test before starting a new exercise program. Talk to your physician about it.

Gear up for success

One of the easiest ways to increase the likelihood that you'll stick with your exercise program is obtaining proper gear. In the case of walking or running, this can be very simple. The most important gear for walkers and runners is proper footwear and clothing. Swimming and water aerobics require a swimsuit, swim goggles, and non-skid water sneakers. In addition to a road or stationary bike in good condition, cyclers need non-chafing clothing and the right shoes for safety.

You can get good advice about walking or running shoes appropriate for your level of fitness, the terrain that you walk or run on, and climatic conditions in which you exercise at any good athletic shoe store. Appropriate, well-fitting footwear increases your comfort during your walk or run and thereby encourages you to stick with your program. For a better fit, buy walking or running shoes during the afternoon because your feet tend to swell a little bit during the day, and you get a better fit in the afternoon.

If you will be walking, running, or cycling out of doors, make sure you have comfortable clothing. Most regular exercisers understand the value of *layering* their exercise clothing. Consider rainy and cold weather clothes, too. Don't forget a hat and gloves.

Get started with a basic 12-week aerobic program

I'm going to assume that you have not been regularly active and start with a basic program that anyone can use. This program, shown in Table 5-1, enables you to start slowly and safely and progress steadily over about 12 weeks to a fitness level that will enable you to engage in lengthier and/or more intense activities. I recommend that you start by walking, even if you plan to use another primary aerobic activity. However, you can adapt this program to swimming or cycling. Your intensity should be moderate for all sessions; after 12 weeks, you can gradually pick up the pace if you wish.

Table 5-1	12-Week Aerobic Activity Starter Program		
Week	**Duration**	**Sessions per Week**	**Activity Days***
Week 1	5 minutes	3 days	M W F
Week 2	6-7 minutes	3 days	M W F
Week 3	8-10 minutes	4 days	M W F S
Week 4	10 minutes	4 days	M W F S
Week 5	10-12 minutes	5 days	M W T S S
Week 6	12-15 minutes	5 days	M W T S S
Week 7	15 minutes	5 days	M T T F S
Week 8	15-20 minutes	5 days	M W T F S
Week 9	20 minutes	5 days	M T T S S
Week 10	20-25 minutes	5 days	M T T F S
Week 11	25 minutes	5 days	T W F S S
Week 12	30 minutes	5 days	M W T S S

* You can put your activity sessions on the days of the week that work best for you, but it's best to schedule rest days within the 5 days.

After you have completed the 12-week program, you should be able to walk, swim, or bicycle at moderate intensity for 30 minutes. If at any time, you feel your effort is too hard, take a 1 to 2 minute break and resume at a slower pace. After 12 weeks, you should also be ready to join more intensive classes or activities such as aerobic dance, zumba, spinning, and running.

 Tracking your activity will help you stay on course. Research shows that people who keep a record of their activity (and diet) tend to stick with the program to reach their goals. You can find a free tracker online at www.choosemyplate.gov; the American Heart Association also provides a free activity tracker at http://www.startwalkingnow.org/mystart_tracker.jsp.

Add strength training

Although strength training has multiple overall benefits, it should be used in conjunction with aerobic activity, not in place of it. Because strength training can cause dramatic increases in blood pressure, if you have high blood pressure or coronary heart disease, you should consult with your doctor and work with a skilled health professional with knowledge and background in cardiac rehabilitation.

Nonetheless, strength training can be useful in reducing your risk of heart disease or in treating heart disease. Strength training can benefit heart patients by increasing the efficiency of their muscles, thus enabling them to carry out either leisure-time or work activities at a lower percentage of their maximal capacity. Regular strength training also can help prevent weight gain, which is of significant benefit for patients with heart disease.

 If you already have heart disease and want to start strength training, or if you want to use strength training to lower your risk of heart disease, the best advice is to find a skilled health professional with training in this area. This person can help you establish the best routine for you.

Sticking with your program for the long haul

Following these five tips can help you stick with your program of accumulating moderate-intensity activities:

✔ **Set a time and place.** Most people find that routines are helpful, so try to establish at least one time and place for physical activity each day. How about walking the dog in the morning or taking a ten-minute, mind-clearing walk at lunch? Enter your activity session in your calendar (I do!).

✔ **Be prepared.** Always be on the lookout for unexpected opportunities to insert a little activity into the nooks and crannies of your life. Adopt a mind-set that emphasizes more physical activity.

✔ **Include family and friends.** Undertaking activities with family and friends makes them more social and enjoyable. Being active regularly as a family also starts your children on the right path for lifelong health. Having friends or family depending on you also increases the likelihood that you'll make time for physical activity each day.

✔ **Have fun.** If your activity isn't fun, you aren't going to do it. Choose things that you look forward to doing.

✔ **Prioritize.** If you don't make physical activity a priority, you're highly unlikely to stay with it day in and day out, week in and week out, month in and month out.

Considering why walking is the best heart-healthy exercise

Extensive research conducted by my laboratory and others demonstrates some simple facts about walking:

✔ Virtually everyone can get aerobic benefit from walking. Walking is particularly suitable for patients with a variety of heart conditions because the intensity is extremely flexible.

✔ Walking is usually the simplest and most convenient form of physical activity for the vast majority of people.

✔ Walking is simple — as easy as putting one foot in front of the other, opening your front door, and setting off down the road.

✔ Most of the research that shows that regular physical activity lowers the risk of heart disease has focused on walking.

✔ For most people, I recommend walking as the best form of regular exercise to lower the risk of cardiovascular disease — and so do 90 percent of my fellow physicians.

If you prefer a different form of physical activity and/or aerobic exercise, however, don't be dismayed. Almost everything I say about walking also applies to other forms of aerobic exercise. All aerobic activities are equally good in terms of their cardiovascular benefits.

Overcoming excuses

Everyone, even the most regular exerciser, faces periods when it is more difficult to exercise. Often, people who want to exercise are their own worst enemies because they make up excuses for not sticking with their exercise programs. Here are some common excuses and how to overcome them:

✔ **Excuse:** I am busy. I don't have time.

Solution: Find a specific time to exercise and put it on your calendar or appointment book. Keep your appointment to exercise the same way you'd keep any other appointment. If your calendar is digital, set an automatic reminder.

✔ **Excuse:** The weather is bad.

Solution: Always have a Plan B. Be ready for bad weather by finding a number of alternative locations for your walking program, such as a shopping mall or a fitness facility. Better yet, buy a treadmill and walk at home. Anticipate changes of season. For example, before the weather turns bitterly cold, be sure to plan where and when you're going to walk during the winter months.

✔ **Excuse:** I am too tired.

Solution: You may be exercising too hard, if it makes you tired, but you may also want to consider exercising earlier in the day. Your walk should invigorate you. If it doesn't, you need to adjust your schedule or the intensity of your walk.

✔ **Excuse:** Walking is boring! I don't look forward to it or enjoy it.

Solution: Vary your walking route. Employ different strategies, such as walking with family and friends. Join a group, such as the local mall-walking group, or walk while listening to music.

✔ **Excuse:** Walking cuts into family time.

Solution: Ask your family members to join in your walking program. That way it benefits everyone!

Making Sure You Don't Overdo It

When it comes to exercise, too much can be hard on your heart and your health. Don't think that's an excuse not to exercise; it's simply a warning that you need to take it slow and keep close tabs on how you feel during and after activity.

Recognizing six signs of overexercising

When starting an exercise program, many people don't realize how easy it is to over-exercise. Watch out for these warning signals:

- **Difficulty finishing:** If you can't complete your exercise program with energy to spare, decrease your pace (intensity) and/or your distance.

- **Inability to carry on a normal conversation while walking:** If you can't talk normally while you exercise, you're going too fast. Slow down!

- **Faintness or nausea after exercising:** If your walking (or other activity) is too intense or you stop walking too abruptly, you can feel faint. This happens because increased blood flow to your legs when you're walking may cause blood to pool temporarily in the veins, making it difficult for the heart to maintain an adequate output. Decrease your walking pace and increase the amount of time you spend cooling down. If you nonetheless feel faint again, see your doctor.

- **Chronic fatigue:** If during the remainder of the day or evening after exercise, you feel tired rather than stimulated, you're exercising too hard. If you feel fatigued or experience chest pain after exercise, decrease the pace and/or distance of your workout. Seeing your doctor also is a good idea.

- **Sleeplessness:** A proper exercise program should make getting a good night's sleep easier, not more difficult. If you're having more difficulty sleeping normally, decrease the amount of exercise you do until your symptoms subside.

- **Increased aches and pains in your joints:** Some muscle discomfort is inevitable when you start exercising after being very inactive. However, your joints should neither hurt nor continue feeling stiff. Make sure that you're warming up and stretching correctly. Muscle cramping and back discomfort also may indicate poor warm-up techniques. If symptoms persist, consult your physician.

Sounding medic alert: Symptoms to watch for during exercise

The key to safe exercise is never leaving your common sense at home. Staying in tune with any symptoms that you have during an exercise session is important for achieving maximum benefit and safety from exercising, especially when you're at risk for heart disease or already have established signs or symptoms or manifestations of heart disease. If the following symptoms occur during exercise, contact your physician before continuing your walking routine or any other form of physical activity:

- **Discomfort in the chest, arm, upper body, neck, or jaw:** These symptoms may very well be angina. If you have any questions, you need to discuss them with your doctor. This type of discomfort may be of any intensity and may be experienced as aching, burning, or a sensation of fullness or tightness.

✓ **Faintness or lightheadedness:** These symptoms may occur after exercise whenever your cool-down is too brief. This situation usually isn't serious and can be managed by extending the cool-down. However, if you experience a fainting spell or feel that you're about to faint during exercise, immediately discontinue the activity and consult your physician.

✓ **Excessive shortness of breath:** While you're walking or performing any other form of aerobic exercise, you can expect the rate and depth of your breathing to increase, but you shouldn't feel uncomfortable. A good rule to follow is that breathing should not be so difficult that talking becomes an effort. If wheezing develops or if recovery from shortness of breath takes more than five minutes at the conclusion of an exercise session, you need to consult with your doctor.

✓ **Irregular pulse:** If your pulse is irregular, skips, or races, either during or after exercise, such that it differs from your normal pulse, consulting your physician is important.

✓ **Changes in usual symptoms:** If your usual symptoms change — an increase in angina or shortness of breath, for example — or pain occurs or becomes more severe or persistent in an arthritic joint or at the site of a previous orthopedic injury, you need to consult with your physician.

✓ **Any other symptoms:** Finally, you always need to discuss any other symptoms that concern you with your physician. Physical activity should be a pleasure and not a chore. Pain is a warning sign that you should never ignore.

Some medications can also affect the intensity of your exercise program but not its effectiveness. Discuss this possibility with your doctor.

Chapter 6

Tapping the Power of the Mind/ Body Connection

The mind, the emotions, and the heart long have been linked in the human imagination. Since prehistoric times, people have identified the heart as the seat of love and other emotions.

- You give your heart to the ones you love.

- When your heart breaks, you suffer *heartache,* which the dictionary defines as "anguish of mind."

- Like medieval knights swearing allegiance to their king, people still place hands over their physical hearts to pledge loyalty to their nations.

- A close call "makes your heart stop" and "scares you to death."

- If you fight bravely to the end in any cause, you "never lose heart," but if you give up easily, you're "fainthearted."

- Anger makes your "blood boil," but a positive, cheerful outlook makes you "lighthearted."

Humankind's prehistoric ancestors undoubtedly used the same telling expressions linking the mind and heart as they told stories around the fire in the family cave or confronted the woolly mammoth outside in the wilderness.

Even though modern science has taken a long time to begin to catch up with folklore and language, scientists are beginning to understand that powerful links between mind and body actually exist. Although emotional states and psychological health appear to have an impact on virtually every organ system, the links between the mind and heart probably have been the most fully studied and understood. In this chapter, I review links between stress, anger, love, friendship, intimacy, fear, and many other physiological states and cardiac health. I also review some simple strategies for controlling stress and anger and opening up your heart to promote cardiac health.

Understanding the Connections between Stress and the Heart

High stress levels constitute one of the cardiac health risks (and general health risks) that everyone faces daily. In fact, a growing body of scientific and medical evidence links stress to a variety of illnesses ranging from heart disease and cancer to the common cold. Unfortunately, stress is pervasive in today's modern, fast-paced society. One study from the National Institute of Mental Health found that more than 30 percent of adults experience enough stress in their daily lives to impair their performance at work or at home.

Defining stress

Despite literally hundreds of studies about stress, a precise definition is frustratingly difficult to come up with. Perhaps the best simple definition came from Canadian scientist Hans Selye, who in 1956 defined stress as "the non-specific response of the body to any demands made on it" in his pioneering book *The Stress of Life*. The *demand* (the thing that stresses you out, be it a traffic jam, power outage, or deadline) and the *response* (your internal reaction to, say, a $2,000 car-repair bill or any other demand) are the key components of stress. No doubt you're faced with many demands (stressors) every day. How you respond is up to you, but remember that the way you respond can contribute either to improved cardiac health or to increased cardiac risk.

Describing positive versus negative stress

Many people don't realize that having positive stress is possible. But a certain amount of stress may be necessary for you to reach your optimal performance. For example, outstanding athletes often perform at their best in the "big game." And you may be one of the many people who work best when faced with a deadline. However, when stress becomes excessive or when your response to the stress becomes negative, your health in general, and your cardiac health in particular, may be harmed.

Linking stress to heart disease

When it comes to the heart, stress can

- ✔ Increase your likelihood of developing coronary heart disease (CHD)
- ✔ Create chest discomfort that can mimic heart disease
- ✔ Cause palpitations or even very serious arrhythmias
- ✔ Contribute to the development of high blood pressure

Numerous scientific studies link job-related stress to an increase in the likelihood of your developing coronary heart disease. Some of these studies show that heart attacks occur more often during the six months following negative life changes, such as divorce, financial setback, or the death of a spouse or close relative than they do during the six months before these negative life changes.

Linking stress to high blood pressure

The link between stress and high blood pressure is well established. Many years ago, Dr. Walter Cannon, a famous physiologist, coined the phrase *fight or flight* to describe the physiological changes that occur during stress. He linked this response to the genetic makeup of humans. When confronted by a dangerous and frightening saber-toothed tiger, for example, ancient human ancestors needed to make an immediate decision whether to stand and fight, freeze with fear, or immediately take flight. One physiological response to this stress is elevated blood pressure.

Unfortunately, people still have the genetic makeup that causes their blood pressure to rise during emotionally stressful situations. For example, studies show that air-traffic controllers, whose jobs place them under continually high levels of stress, are more likely to have high blood pressure than people in many other professions.

Constant pressure caused by events and situations over which you feel you have only minimal control is a particularly dangerous form of stress. For example, blood pressure rises in soldiers during times of war, in civilians faced with natural disasters, such as floods or explosions, and in entire societies in which social order is unstable.

Linking Type A personality traits to heart problems

About 50 years ago, Dr. Ray Rosenman and Dr. Meyer Friedman developed the concept of *Type A Personality,* which links certain kinds of behavior and personality traits with an increased incidence of heart attack. Unfortunately, the concept of Type A behavior often is loosely and incorrectly applied to any hard-driving, busy worker.

The research defines Type A behavior, however, as containing aggression, competitiveness, and hostility. Individuals who exhibit true Type A behavior also are likely to have a sense of incredible urgency as they attempt to accomplish poorly defined goals in the shortest period of time. Likewise, they often are angry when confronted with unexpected delays. The combination of *frustration* and *anger* is essential to manifest the cardiac danger associated with a Type A personality. Hard workers who are happy in their work, even when they're workaholics, are more likely to fall into what Rosenman and Friedman characterized as *Type B personalities* and are not at increased risk of heart disease.

Linking anger to dangerous heart problems

More recent studies from a variety of investigators, including Dr. Redford Williams at Duke University, show that the hostility component of Type A behavior specifically accounts for almost all the increased risk of cardiac disease. Using one of the subscales on psychological inventories administered to many participants in large heart-health trials, Dr. Williams and his colleagues identified cynical mistrust of others, frequent experience of angry feelings, and overt expression of cynicism and anger in aggressive behavior as key factors that make up the psychological profile that increases the risk of developing heart disease. In real-life situations, this discovery points not only to the knowledge that anger kills when you let it control your behavior — think road rage — but also to the knowledge that it may also kill by damaging your heart.

Making Connections: Friendship, Intimacy, and Cardiac Health

People who have trouble connecting with others and developing intimate relationships also may have a higher risk of developing heart disease and suffering its consequences. The opposite also is true: Those who have strong relationships with others also have a healthier heart.

Suffering the lonely heart

Maybe poets are absolutely correct when they write about dying of a broken heart. Numerous studies show that individuals who feel isolated and alone are much more likely to experience health problems, including heart disease and cancer, than are individuals who experience intimacy, love, and a sense of being connected. Take a look at the findings:

- The prestigious *New England Journal of Medicine* published a study of more than 2,300 men who had survived a heart attack. The risk of death for participants who were classified as socially isolated and having a high degree of stress was more than four times that of participants with low levels of stress and isolation. These relationships held up even when the study was controlled for other cardiac risk factors, such as smoking, diet, exercise, and weight.

- In a Duke University study of 1,400 men and women who had blockage of at least one coronary artery (determined by coronary angiography), study participants who weren't married and didn't have at least one close confidant were more than three times more likely to have died at follow-up than participants who were married and/or had a confidant.

- In a third study, participants who suffered a recent heart attack and lived alone experienced twice the risk of dying after a heart attack when compared with participants who lived with one or more other individuals and described their relationships as close.

In many other studies conducted in diverse cultures, social isolation has been found to increase the risk of heart disease, sudden death, and cancer.

Promoting the healing power of love

Numerous studies show that people who give and receive love actually decrease their risks of heart disease and other diseases. Check out these examples:

- In one famous study conducted among Harvard undergraduates in the early 1950s, participants were asked to describe their relationships with their parents. When their medical records were examined in the 1980s, the results were astounding. Ninety-one percent of these former students who said they didn't have a loving relationship with their parents had been diagnosed with serious diseases by midlife, most prominently CHD and high blood pressure. However, fewer than 50 percent of the participants who reported warm and loving relationships with their parents had developed these chronic diseases in adult life.

✔ A similar study conducted at Johns Hopkins Medical School shows that physician participants who ultimately developed severe medical problems were much less likely to have described close loving relationships earlier in life than were participants who had not suffered such medical problems.

✔ In yet another study of elderly individuals with heart disease, participants who were able to reach out for help had one-third the risk of dying from heart disease as older individuals who tried to go it alone.

Connecting for heart health

As you can see, the ability to connect with other individuals appears to carry significant cardiac benefit. If you feel isolated or lonely, it may be time to make some connections by

✔ Investing time and thought in friends and/or family as seriously as you do in your work.

✔ Joining an interest group. From chess clubs to gardening clubs, book clubs to folkdance societies, running clubs to writing classes, an activity-related group that matches your interests is out there for you to benefit from.

✔ Finding a third place. Beyond home and work, people long have benefited from a close connection to a *third place* in their communities. For many it's their church, synagogue, mosque, or temple. For others, it's a social group, community organization, or other activity or group that is meaningful to them. The identity of your third place isn't as important as the fact that you have one.

Being "Scared to Death" and Other Mind/Body Links

Everybody has experienced a racing heart — after a bad scare or an angry moment, for instance. Strong emotion also can produce serious rhythm disturbances (see Chapter 2).

Understanding that mind/body links are hardwired

Although feelings of joy, anger, or depression may be complex functions, your body has only a limited vocabulary of physiological responses to them. Most of these responses are mediated through the nervous system, which controls all your body's functions.

The nervous system is divided into two major branches: the *sympathetic nervous system* and the *parasympathetic nervous system.*

✔ When the sympathetic nervous system (the part of the nervous system that results in the fight or flight response) is stimulated, various rhythm disturbances caused by rapid heartbeat or extra beats can occur. Fear and anger are two stimuli that trigger this system. Stress can also cause palpitations that typically are experienced by individuals as skipped heartbeats or irregular heartbeats.

✔ When the parasympathetic nervous system (the part of the nervous system that is responsible for maintenance of routine body function, also called *rest and digest functions*) is stimulated, a slow heart rate can result. The most common result of an excessively slow heartbeat is fainting. Typically any condition that produces a faint — crowded room, hot day, having blood drawn — triggers this system.

People who are more susceptible to rhythm abnormalities provoked by emotion also are more likely to have underlying cardiac disease. But occasionally people with normal coronary arteries develop severe cardiac arrhythmias in stressful settings.

"Dropping dead" from stress — myth or reality?

Plenty of anecdotal evidence points to the fact that people may collapse and die when faced with sudden overwhelming emotional stress. Dr. George Engel, a leading researcher in this area, reviewed a number of cases in which psychological stress appeared to cause sudden death. He found that sudden death commonly took place during one of the following events:

✔ Hearing of the death of a friend or relative

✔ Suffering an acute episode of grief

✔ Mourning a sad event or its anniversary

✔ Losing status or self-esteem

✔ Experiencing personal threat or danger

✔ Experiencing a reunion or triumph

Specific evidence often is lacking in these situations, but experts believe that in most of these circumstances the sudden death results from a severe form of cardiac arrhythmia called *ventricular tachycardia,* which ultimately degenerates into a fatal cardiac arrhythmia called *ventricular fibrillation,* where the heart ineffectively quivers and is unable to pump out blood.

Sudden stress, such as the death of a loved one, can also cause a condition that mimics a heart attack; it is known as *broken-heart syndrome, Takastubo syndrome*, or *Takastubo cardiomyopathy*. The sudden surge of stress hormones temporarily weakens the left ventricle muscles, disrupting the heart's normal pumping and causing symptoms that mimic a heart attack. This relatively rare condition occurs more commonly in women than men. Although it rarely causes death or lasting problems, like an actual heart attack, this condition requires quick diagnosis and treatment.

Understanding stress caused by heart problems

In much the same way that psychological stress can result in either acute or chronic heart problems, the flip side is also true — heart disease can result in psychological problems.

The period *after* a heart attack has drawn the most attention from researchers. Many people go through a three-part psychological response to having a heart attack that includes

- ✔ Initially experiencing great anxiety produced by the physical event of heart attack and by fear of dying.

- ✔ Denying that you've had a heart attack or denying that anything is seriously wrong with you.

- ✔ Settling into what is known as *homecoming depression*. In this situation, you may become depressed and worried about the long-term consequences of your heart attack or become remorseful about lifestyle practices that may have contributed to your cardiac problem.

During and after a heart attack, psychological stress typically diminishes when the patient is surrounded by caring, supportive healthcare workers and family. Studies show that individuals who have such strong support systems are much more likely to recover from a heart attack than individuals who do not.

Understanding the heart attack that isn't: Heart disease mimics

Studies show that 10 percent to 20 percent of cardiac patients may have symptoms caused not by their heart disease but instead by underlying emotional disorders. Perhaps an equal number of individuals who don't have heart disease visit their physicians with manifestations of underlying emotional problems that may initially be confused with heart disease. The three most common emotional disorders that can mimic heart disease are

- ✔ **Anxiety states:** The spectrum of anxiety states extends from chronic anxiety through attacks of anxiety in specific settings. Such anxiety states often may be accompanied by rapid heartbeat, palpitations, chest pain, or tightness or shortness of breath. Although these symptoms need to be taken seriously, a physician typically can rule out serious cardiac disease. Anxiety states typically respond well to support and reassurance, including psychological counseling and therapy whenever necessary.

- ✔ **Panic disorder:** Although panic disorder is one of the anxiety states, its presentation may be so dramatic and so similar to cardiovascular disease that it deserves separate consideration. Individuals with panic disorder can experience a sudden outpouring of feelings of terror and impending doom. These may be accompanied by chest pain, severe shortness of breath, and irregular heartbeat — symptoms that may resemble serious cardiac disease. Attacks often occur in predictable settings, such as crowded rooms, theaters, or other public places where exit may be restricted. A physician typically can distinguish between a panic disorder and serious heart disease. Taking a careful history is important to making the right diagnosis.

- ✔ **Depression:** Considerable overlap exists between depression and heart disease. Sometimes people who have heart disease become depressed, and in other instances, medicines used to treat high blood pressure or CHD tend to have side effects that may cause depression. Treatment of the underlying depression typically resolves all symptoms in such cases.

Understanding how psychotropic medications may affect the heart

Psychotropic medications act on the mind (*psyche* = mind; *tropic* = influencing) and often are prescribed for anxiety or for depression. Psychotropic medications have made it easier to manage these conditions effectively, and they are prescribed for large numbers of people. However, many medications that work on the brain may also affect the heart. For example, some medicines used for treating depression may contribute to rapid heartbeat and palpitations.

If you suffer from depression, taking your medication is important, and most antidepressant medications are safe. But if you also have heart disease, you may want to discuss with your doctor any potential side effects taking any of these medicines may have on the heart.

Keeping Stress and Anger at Bay

Do you get bent out of shape when the weather ruins your plans? When a driver cuts you off? When a last-minute project keeps you late at work? If you do, you're risking serious damage to your heart, which can stand up to only so much stress and anger. Reducing these risk factors is up to you, and it's not as hard as you may think.

Controlling stress with a four-part plan

Stress may be dangerous for the heart, but the good news is that some simple strategies may significantly lower stress and thereby improve cardiac health. Here are four ways to lower the stress in your life and contribute to cardiac health:

✔ **Modify or eliminate circumstances that contribute to stress and cardiac symptoms.** People often simply do not realize that aspects of their daily lives can compound problems with stress. Cutting back on coffee, tea, energy drinks, and other caffeinated beverages, for example, may make a substantial difference in your stress levels and manifestations like cardiac palpitations. Fatigue and insomnia may also contribute to stress, so be sure that you get plenty of rest and a good night's sleep whenever you're experiencing symptoms of stress. You also need to avoid the temptation to use alcohol as a way to relax. Although it may seem to offer a temporary release from stress, it usually leads to greater problems.

✔ **Live in the present.** The basis for all effective stress reduction is being able to live in the present. It may sound simple, but many people spend an inordinate amount of time either regretting the past or fearing the future. Strategies such as biofeedback, visualization, and medications can help you live in the present and substantially lower stress levels.

✔ **Get out of your own way.** Many people compound the inevitable stresses of their daily lives by layering on negative feelings concerning these stresses. Recognizing that no one can live a life that is completely free of stress is as important as trying not to compound the problem by allowing feelings of negativity or low self-worth to make stress worse.

✔ **Develop a personal plan for stress.** Developing a personal plan to alleviate stress is one of the most effective ways to handle it on an ongoing basis, instead of allowing it to become free-floating anxiety. Many people find that daily exercise, meditation, taking a timeout (either alone or with family), and other such strategies provide effective ways of controlling the stresses of daily life.

Ten-minute timeouts against stress

"Step away for ten a day": Short, calming breaks from your daily routine can lower your stress dramatically. Try one of these techniques:

Go outside. The right short break outside can ease the tension.

> *Do:* Stroll. Clear your mind. Smell the flowers. People watch.

> *Don't:* Think about your schedule. Outline that memo. Pick at a worry.

Tune into calm. You can also get away right in your office or easy chair. Simply find a quiet, comfortable spot. Allow no interruptions. Sit quietly and focus on becoming calm. Consciously clear your mind, gently pushing away any intruding thoughts of work or problems. Listening to quiet music, visualizing peaceful scenes, or focusing on deep, slow breathing may help. A luxurious stretch at the end of your ten minutes can be a nice transition back to activity.

Listen to your body. Using biofeedback techniques can help you foster a relaxed state. In research conducted in my laboratory, I found that people who take ten minutes each day to focus on relaxing were able to dramatically reduce their stress levels. They used the same techniques that I described earlier, but they also relied on a heart-rate monitor as their point of focus. Sitting quietly, focus on your heart rate and imagine it going lower. Using the other visualization techniques in combination with biofeedback can enhance your ten-minute timeout.

Meditate. Practicing any of several formal types of meditation can be useful to anyone who enjoys it. *Meditation For Dummies* (Wiley) can get you started.

Catnap. If you're one of those lucky souls who can drop instantly to sleep and wake refreshed in 10 or 15 minutes, you can experience the ten-minute timeout in one of its most satisfying forms (at least, so say its devotees).

Controlling anger with five simple steps

The hostility or anger component of the Type A personality poses the most significant cardiac risk. Here are five simple strategies for helping you control anger:

- ✔ **Learn how to trust other people.** An open heart is a healthy heart. Individuals who are isolated and fearful of other people increase their risk of cardiac disease. By making an effort to open yourself up to trusting other individuals, you can substantially lower your risk of heart disease.

- ✔ **Plant a garden and care for a pet.** The Irish poet William Butler Yeats said the definition of a civilized human being is one who plants a garden and cares for a domestic pet. This concept is not only a prescription for a civilized human being, but also a prescription for a heart-healthy life.

- **Practice asserting yourself.** Many people keep their emotions bottled up inside. They're often pleasantly surprised to find out that by standing up for what they believe (in a pleasant way, of course), they can control unwarranted stress in their lives and lead a happier daily existence.

- **Become a volunteer.** A wonderful body of literature suggests that volunteers not only do good for other people, but they also improve their own health. Somehow, the act of giving of yourself to other people results in improved health for yourself.

- **Practice forgiveness.** Many people keep themselves in a constant state of anger for wrongs or supposed slights from other people or from the world at large. Learning how to forgive others is one of the very best things that you can do to improve your own cardiac health. While you're at it, forgive yourself, too, for past shortcomings — imagined or real.

Tap the calm of yoga and tai chi

Would you like to improve your flexibility, balance, muscle, and core strength while reducing stress and increasing relaxation? Then try one or both of these ancient (and proven) techniques that truly tap the power of the mind/body connection.

Hatha yoga (not one of the new "power" varieties) uses poses, breathing, and meditation to help practitioners achieve physical and mental benefits. This gentle and relatively low-intensity activity can help reduce blood pressure and stress levels.

Tai chi has been called "meditation in motion." Moving slowly through the exercises of tai chi helps you focus in the present and release tension and anxiety while the low-intensity exercises strengthen balance and upper and lower body muscles as well as bone strength. As videos of Asian elders indicate, tai chi is appropriate throughout the lifespan.

Chapter 7

Taking a Family Approach to Preventing Heart Disease

Home is where the heart is. That familiar sentiment also sets up another insight: Home is where heart health starts. Practices and habits that children develop early in life are the ones that they typically continue to follow in adult life. Research has long shown that the first manifestations of adult atherosclerosis often start in childhood. By the same token, heart-healthy habits learned in childhood can lead to a lifetime of reduced risk of heart disease and other chronic diseases. As parents, then, you can do a lot to set your children on the path to lifelong health not only by the healthy behaviors you help them develop but also by the way you model those behaviors in your own lives.

In an ideal world, perfectly healthy parents would raise perfectly healthy children. But the world is never ideal. If you are reading this book, the chances are that you or someone you love has a diagnosis of one or more risk factors for heart disease, including coronary heart disease (CHD) itself. In that case, home is where you look first for support. Spouses ought to be able to count on each other as first allies in any heath challenge; that support, research shows, can make a tremendous positive difference. Challenges also tend to increase as people grow older. At that point, vital support again starts with family.

But just how can family members support each other for better heart health and overall well-being at each life stage? In this chapter, I provide some tips and techniques that research studies and clinical experience have found effective.

Achieving heart health is a lifelong endeavor. And everyone has the most success when the whole family succeeds in adopting heart-healthy daily practices and habits. As the Sisters Sledge sang, "We are family" and we're giving "love in the family dose." If you haven't already, taking the first steps to engage your family in heart-healthy eating and activity patterns will be giving that love in a family dose.

Setting Your Children on the Path to a Heart-Healthy Future

Fostering healthy habits in your children sets them up for a healthy future. Not just heart health but general overall health will result from first understanding why it is important to help children develop heart-healthy practices and then taking proven steps to teach them how to make heart-healthy choices.

Understanding that risk of heart disease starts very early

Many risk factors play a role in the complex process that leads to atherosclerosis (as I describe in Chapters 2 and 3). Although most people with atherosclerosis are middle-aged or older before they get a diagnosis of heart disease or experience signs such as angina, many children and adolescents actually have the fatty streaks and fibrous plaques that are the first manifestations of atherosclerosis and that eventually lead to coronary heart disease (CHD). Because they can't be detected by most tests, these early manifestations are called *subclinical*.

Finding early signs of atherosclerosis in children

Evidence that subclinical atherosclerosis begins in childhood first came to light in the early 20th century, when autopsies on young soldiers (most 18 to 20 years old) showed fatty streaks and plaques in the aorta and coronary arteries. Since that time more studies, such as the Bogalusa Heart Study and the PDAY Study (Pathobiological Determinants of Atherosclerosis in Youth), have confirmed these early signs of atherosclerosis in children as young as two years old. Some studies suggest that infants in the womb whose mothers have cholesterol problems may have some fatty streaks in their arteries.

The Bogalusa Heart Study which followed a very large group of individuals from age 2 through age 38 puts these findings into perspective. In more than 200 study participants who died from various causes, autopsies found fatty streaks in the coronary arteries of 50 percent of children aged 2 to 15 and in the arteries of 85 percent of young adults, aged 21 to 39. More extensive fibrous plaques, increasing with age, were observed in 8 percent of the 2- to 15-year-olds and 69 percent of the young adults aged 26 to 39.

Children and youth at greatest risk are those who are overweight or obese and inactive. These factors contribute to a clustering of risk factors such as the following: lipid (fat in the blood) problems, including higher total cholesterol and LDL cholesterol; more insulin resistance (prediabetes); and higher blood pressure. A child who has type 1 diabetes is also at increased risk.

Checking up on potential risk factors in children

Because children develop risk factors for chronic disease, including heart disease, when should your child's regular checkups start including tests for such factors as high blood pressure or cholesterol problems?

Guidelines from the American Academy of Pediatrics recommend that all children should have their blood cholesterol levels checked once between ages 9 and 11 and then once again between ages 17 and 21. If your family has a history of high cholesterol *(hypercholesterolemia),* then your children should have their cholesterol levels checked before age 5. Your pediatrician will then recommend how often after to have cholesterol checked.

Very few children have high blood pressure, but some do. Your pediatrician will begin to check blood pressure when a child is about 3. The doctor will take into account the child's age, gender, and height to evaluate the readings appropriate for your child.

Because many potential risk factors in childhood are related to being overweight (and inactive), the most important thing parents can do for children is to make heart-healthy patterns of eating and activity a part of your family's lifestyle from the beginning. Your child's pediatrician will evaluate your child's weight at each checkup. Adjustments in diet and amount of activity usually help children easily stay within a healthy weight range. If there are problems, discuss these with the pediatrician.

Modeling heart-healthy behaviors makes a difference for children

One of the most important things (if not the most important) that parents can do to raise healthy children who develop healthy habits is to model positive behaviors. The home environment you provide is also important. For example, the children of parents who encourage them to eat well and to get plenty of exercise and who model those healthful behaviors themselves tend to have more heart-healthy habits and lower risks for chronic disease.

"Do what I say, not what I do!" This admonition, as every parent knows, may be among the most useless on the planet. If you want to help your children make daily choices and develop habits that foster heart health (and overall health) for life, you must model those choices and behaviors yourself. Your child is not going to gobble up at least five fruits and vegetables daily if you are only wolfing down potatoes five ways, for example. Sending children outdoors to "play" while you settle in front of the television or computer screen wastes your breath. You get the picture. Research indicates that parental influence is most effective when you walk the walk, not just talk the talk.

Providing a home environment that makes it easy for children to make healthy choices is also important. For example, having fresh fruit and other nutritious snacks easily available on a countertop and in the pantry encourages their consumption. Similarly, you need to provide opportunities and encouragement for active play. Something as simple as providing toys, such as balls, trikes or bicycles, and swing sets, for outside play and making sure there is a safe outside space for play can encourage children to be active. When homes, such as apartments, have no space for outside play, parents may need to prioritize taking children to playgrounds and parks or finding afterschool and weekend programs that provide safe environments for study and recreation. Many community centers and schools and organizations such as Boys and Girls Clubs offer such options.

A final aspect of modeling healthful behaviors involves including children in planning and creating healthy activities. These range from encouraging kids to help with buying healthy foods and creating tasty meals with those foods to involving them in planning family and personal physical activities.

Fostering nutritious food choices and eating habits

Children must grow in their ability to enjoy a wide range of foods just as they have to develop in other areas of life. As any parent or caretaker of young children knows, most infants don't like sour or bitter foods. (Much research suggests that human beings are born with preferences for sweet and salty foods over bitter or sour foods. The hypothesis is that, in the prehistoric past, sweet and salty foods were more likely to be safe to eat.) Unfortunately, many foods like vegetables that are most nutritious may fall into the "bitter" or "not sweet" category for toddler taste buds. Extensive research has identified a number of opportunities and techniques to encourage children in their first five years and beyond to develop healthful eating habits:

> ✔ **Eat healthful foods during pregnancy and breastfeeding.** What pregnant mothers-to-be and breastfeeding moms eat may influence children's acceptance of certain foods. Interestingly, research suggests that children of women who eat foods such as garlic, cumin, curry, and even

carrot juice, all of which have compounds or "flavors" detectable in amniotic fluid or breast milk, may predispose children to like or accept such foods when they start eating solid foods.

✔ **Present new foods to children multiple times — 5 to 15 times.** Most young children tend to reject new foods when they first encounter them. After one or two rejections, many parents quit offering the food to the child. Research suggests, however, that you need to offer a new food to a child at least 5 times, and perhaps as many as 10 to 15 times, before the child makes the food a part of his or her regular, accepted foods. Children also associate food with its social context; so seeing parents and older siblings enjoying foods can encourage young children to try them.

✔ **Don't use food as a reward or punishment.** Is there an adult who does not remember being told, "Eat your vegetables or you can't have any dessert"? Not many, probably. However, it turns out that this popular parental technique is actually counterproductive for most children. Using a popular food as a reward for eating an rejected food (such as green vegetables) or as a punishment for "bad" or unacceptable behavior (such as not trying green vegetables) tends to reinforce the child's negative feelings about and rejection of the nonpreferred food. The same principle holds for using food as a reward or withholding food as a punishment for other misbehaviors.

✔ **Make nutritious snacks easily available. Don't stock empty-calorie snacks in your pantry.** In my family, we always keep a bowl of fresh fruit, washed and ready-to-eat, on a kitchen counter that everyone can reach. Fruit needing refrigeration is ready in a designated spot in the refrigerator. And here's a good technique for whole grain snacks: package dry whole-grain cereal, crackers, and the like in single-serving reusable containers in a designated spot in the pantry. Label allowable servings — even 2-year-olds can understand "one per afternoon" even though they can't read the label.

✔ **Eat together as a family as often as possible.** Research shows that in families that frequently eat breakfast and/or dinner together, both children and teens tend to have more nutritious eating patterns and maintain more healthful body weights than those who don't. Meals together also provide a social context for families to share with each other, which fosters a supportive environment.

✔ **Work with your child's preschool and school to provide healthy nutrition.** In most families today (two parent or single parent), the adults work fulltime. As a result, children eat more meals away from home than they did several decades ago. The content of those foods and portion sizes are not typically in your parental control, but where possible work with the schools to encourage making healthful food practices a priority. In many places, if you are not satisfied with the school's meal or snack offerings, your child has the option of bringing a lunch and/or snack from home. Always work together with older children to manage this option so that they buy into the plan.

- ✔ **Limit screen time.** A number of population studies show that the more time children, youth, or adults spend in front of a television or computer screen or playing video games, the more likely they are to overeat or to eat energy-dense foods and the more likely they are to be overweight. Controlled trials show that eating meals or snacking (often right out of the bag) while watching television or playing video games or using the computer typically results in people eating more calories.

- ✔ **Involve kids in shopping for and planning and preparing meals.** One of the best ways to get even young children to try new foods is to help them learn about various foods and participate in choosing which to try. The same goes for trying new dishes. Even preschoolers, properly supervised, can help prepare selected dishes. A colleague of mine loves the memory of her 5-year-old niece standing on a stool (adult standing beside her), painstakingly slicing green peppers or cucumbers for salad. Who wouldn't eat a salad she helped prepare? Plus the little girl knew that using a knife was a big "grown up" privilege and she earlier had practiced hard with a plastic knife and soft cheese to learn how to use a knife; she never violated the rule to use a knife only with an adult helping. Now grown with children of her own, that young woman is an outstanding vegetarian cook, whose meals delight family and friends. You don't have to go that extreme to engage your children in planning and preparing healthy dishes and meals they will want to eat.

Encouraging physical activity

Physical activity and exercise are so important to health and physical development for children and adolescents that the Physical Activity Guidelines for Americans 2008 recommends that children and youth get at least 60 minutes of moderate to vigorous physical activity every day. The guidelines also recommend that on at least three days a week, activities include muscle-strengthening and bone-strengthening activities. Several proven strategies can help you enable and encourage your children to be active.

- ✔ **Focus on fun.** Moving your body can be exhilarating. Just watch how toddlers run about the family room or lawn laughing and showing off their new mobility skills. There's no reason for your children (or you) to lose that sense of fun and pleasure as you grow older. As you encourage your children to be active, remember that enjoyment is the first principle.

- ✔ **Play with your children.** Being active with your children is a great way to help them make daily activity a habit. It's also a great way to strengthen your connection with them. Time-honored backyard games work for a wide range of ages; examples include tag, hide-and-seek, tumbling, statues (freeze tag, red light/green light), red rover, steal the bacon, duck duck goose, kickball, soccer, football, playing catch or Frisbee, hacky sack, whiffle ball, corn hole (beanbag toss), badminton, and volleyball. Your kids don't know these games? Teach them. You don't know these games? Google them!

✔ **Make activity an everyday thing.** Take a family walk or bike ride after dinner. Walk with children to school. Go swimming at the community pool or hiking at a local trail on one day per week. Have your child walk the dog with you. Give every family member a pedometer and see who gets the most steps in a week; top stepper gets to select the next family activity outing.

✔ **Turn household chores into activity time.** Turn up the music and boogie while everyone helps out dusting, sweeping, vacuuming, and cleaning. Rake leaves together. Garden together; let each child select a special decorative or edible plant to plant and care for in the garden.

✔ **Plan regular active family events.** Aim for weekly family outings that are active. Hike in a nearby state park or forest. Go geocaching, a popular outdoor treasure hunt adventure. Check out the zoo or a museum or take in a street fair — all activities that require walking. Go fly kites. Try kayaking or canoeing. Go sledding when there's snow.

✔ **Encourage and enable children to try a variety of activities.** Professionals specializing in children's physical activity and exercise note that it is normal for children to try a number of different activities. One day a 12-year-old, for instance, may want to be an Olympic runner and two weeks later an extreme skateboarder or a baseball player. Rather than a drawback, it's good for children and youth to try many different activities. Exploring different activities provides another opportunity for family involvement.

✔ **Help each child match his or her interests with individual sports or activities.** Just because you think your child shows promise at basketball or soccer doesn't mean that he or she will choose and enjoy that sport. Some children latch on early to a team sport such as baseball, swimming, or soccer and stick with it from then on because they enjoy it. Others will participate for a time and then want to switch to another activity. Some children never feel comfortable with competitive team or individual sports. The goal of every parent ought to be to help each child find the activities that he or she enjoys. For example, children who feel physically awkward or don't enjoy competition may enjoy more individual activities and sports such as martial arts, yoga, dance, bicycling, or hiking. Sports that can be competitive can be practiced individually for fun; these include activities such as running, swimming, skating, fencing, and tennis in addition to those just mentioned.

✔ **Practice safety.** Whatever activity your child or your family undertakes, make sure that you have and use the appropriate safety equipment and techniques. Make sure your kids have proper safety equipment for specific activities and know the safety rules. Model those behaviors yourself. I can't begin to count the times that I have seen families out bicycling — the children are all wearing helmets and the parents are bareheaded. I want to shout to them, "Helmets save lives! Put yours on now!"

✔ **Encourage physical education and activity breaks at our child's school.** Children spend a large portion of their weekdays as preschool and school. Even though research shows that getting physical activity during the school day helps students perform better in the classroom, many school districts have cut out physical education (PE) classes and/or activity breaks (recess). Consider ways you can engage with your children's schools and the responsible administrators to express your support for PE and activity as part of the curriculum and school day.

Supporting Your Spouse or Partner in Achieving Heart Health

The realization that you have significant risk factors for heart disease or the diagnosis of heart disease typically comes in adulthood. The most commons risks (see Chapter 3) that arise in the middle years include cholesterol problems, high blood pressure, overweight or obesity, and insulin resistance (pre-diabetes) or type 2 diabetes. Eating a heart-healthy diet and getting adequate regular physical activity are the two most important lifestyle "therapies" that you can use to reduce most of these risks. Having social support, however, is also very important in helping you achieve success in these areas.

For adults who are married or in a committed relationship, the most important social support is usually your spouse or partner. So here are some insights to keep in mind as both of you work toward better health.

✔ **Recognize you are in it together.** Almost all adults Americans have one or more risk factors for heart disease and other chronic conditions. So chances are good that even if it's your significant other, and not you, that has the primary diagnosis, you also probably need to work on adopting healthier lifestyle practices.

✔ **Offer positive support.** Research confirms that providing positive support, rather than critical or ambivalent support, is more likely to help your spouse comply with his or her therapy and to have better heart health. Positive support means doing whatever it takes to enable your partner to carry out the prescribed activities and treatments.

One of the best things you can do is to see that "his/her" diet and "his/her" activity program become "our" diet and "our" activity program. In fact, you'll be glad you did because your health will improve also. This book provides supportive diet and activity strategies you both can use.

Also listen and hear: Communicate with your spouse and respond positively and supportively. Sometimes just feeling like you've been listened to and hearing (out loud!) that someone really cares is really helpful and uplifting. Praise or positive comment on achievements, even small ones, is also usually welcome.

✔ **Don't police behavior.** No matter how hard it is to avoid, don't become a behavior police officer. Trying to monitor every bite your spouse takes, keeping a checklist on activity sessions, or insisting on seeing the results of every blood pressure check or blood sugar reading is counterproductive.

✔ **Enjoy exploring new opportunities together.** What's on your bucket list — the things you and your spouse want to do together and those you're interested in individually? Planning and doing some of these things together can enrich your friendship and supportive togetherness.

Building a Supportive Community for Older Family Members

For most people, growing older comes with the growing occurrence of health problems, including heart disease. Growing older for many people also means that their network of social support is smaller; many people are less able to get about and depend increasingly on family members. At present, according to the Family Caregiver Alliance, approximately 44 million Americans (age 18 and over) provide unpaid assistance to older individuals and adults with disabilities who still live at home and not in a care facility.

If you are providing care for an older family member or friend, caregiving has an impact not only on the health of those you are caring for, but also on your health. If you are an aging adult, then you need to think about the potential support you will need in the future and what the implications are for your children or younger relatives. Whether you are a potential caregiver or person needing care, you should take steps to ensure the best outcomes for those you care about and for yourself. These are just a few tips:

✔ **Educate yourself.** Knowing as much as you can about your parent's or relative's condition will enhance your ability to be supportive. Internet resources such as MedlinePlus.gov and mayoclinic.org provide reliable information on many conditions as well as links to other resources. If you are the older parent or relative needing care, share information that your physicians have provided.

Although giving support may start with something simple like transportation to healthcare appointments, the need for younger family members' support typically increases with time as a parent or relative gets older or possibly sicker. Over the long run, caregiving can pose stress and health risks for caregivers. So if you are younger, start learning about being a caregiver now; http://www.caregiver.org from the Family Caregiver Alliance is an excellent place to start. If you are older, perhaps you have been a caregiver and know something of the demands or you too can learn more about caregiving. Knowing more can help everyone communicate.

✔ **Communicate and build a partnership.** The best approach to supporting your aging parents is to talk honestly about what kind of support they need. You and your siblings should have this conversation with your parents while they are still functionally independent and before a crisis occurs. If you are an older adult or couple, initiate the conversation. Everyone needs to share as honestly as possible about what needs may arise and what each individual can provide. Be realistic and let your heads take charge, not your emotions or fears.

✔ **Get the paperwork done.** If you are a parent or older relative, you owe it to your children or younger relatives to have a will. You also need a durable power of attorney for healthcare and a durable power of attorney for finances, in case you become mentally incapacitated. Be sure that the person(s) who have your powers of attorney have copies of the necessary documents and that all your children know the arrangements you have set up. If you are children of older parents who have not executed these documents, initiate a conversation with your parent(s) about getting this task done.

✔ **Support independence as far as possible.** Most older adults want to be independent and to manage their own affairs and live on their own — not just until they can't "manage" but right up to the end of life.

As a caregiver, being supportive doesn't mean taking command of someone else's life; it means enabling them to do as much as possible for themselves. For a mentally sharp older adult who has physical limitations, that may mean helping primarily with activities that require functional fitness, such as transportation, grocery shopping, housecleaning, and/or assistance with cooking and personal care (or seeing that such assistance is available). For individuals with cognitive decline, supporting independence may mean a different kind of encouragement and help. If you are an older adult who wants to continue being independent, then the first step in showing that independence and family leadership is to do some of the planning I've just described.

✔ **Explore other sources of support.** Many caregivers get worn out because they do not know what other sources of support are available or assume that such services are not affordable. Local, state, and national governments typically have agencies that provide information about services for seniors. The U.S. Administration on Aging (`http://www.aoa.gov`) is a good place to begin your search.

Part III
Tackling Key Health Risks for Heart Disease

Five Foods to Help Lower Blood Pressure and Cholesterol

- **Oats:** Eating a daily serving of oatmeal or ready-to-eat whole grain oat cereal can help lower both blood pressure and overall cholesterol and LDL cholesterol (the bad guys). Beta-glucan, a type of soluble fiber found in oats, gives oats much of their heart health benefits.

- **Olive oil:** Extra virgin olive oil is a mainstay of the Mediterranean Diet, a way of eating associated with heart health. As a rich source of monounsaturated fats, olive oil promotes lower LDL cholesterol levels. Research studies show that regular use of virgin olive oil also results in lower blood pressure for many people.

- **Beans:** Dried beans and other legumes are a good source of soluble fiber, antioxidants, calcium, and other vitamins and minerals that promote healthy blood pressure and lower total and LDL cholesterol and triglyceride levels. They are also a good vegetable source of protein.

- **Dark green vegetables:** Cruciferous vegetables such as leafy, dark greens (collards, spinach, kale, turnip greens, mustard) and broccoli, brussels sprouts, cabbage, and cauliflower are good sources of fiber, antioxidants, calcium, potassium, and other vitamins and minerals. Research shows they help lower cholesterol, fight inflammation, and control blood pressure.

- **Berries:** Strawberries, raspberries, blueberries, and blackberries are rich sources of antioxidants and other micronutrients. Studies show that eating a few berries daily helps to raise good HDL cholesterol and helps to decrease blood pressure. Many other fruits, such as citrus fruits, have different antioxidants that also promote blood pressure, cholesterol, and heart health.

Find out how to enjoy dining out without going high salt or high fat at www.dummies.com/extras/preventingreversingheartdisease.

In this part . . .

✔ Get a grip on what you need to know to control two conditions that are major contributing causes of heart disease: high blood pressure and elevated cholesterol.

✔ Discover proven weight-management techniques that can help you lower your weight and multiple risk factors for heart disease.

✔ Quit smoking by using proven strategies and helpful resources.

Chapter 8

Combating High Blood Pressure

High blood pressure, or *hypertension,* is quite common in the United States. About one-third of the adult population — more than 67 million people — suffer from high blood pressure. Furthermore, as you grow older, you're more likely to have high blood pressure. At some point, almost everyone will develop high blood pressure. But don't despair. You fortunately can take great strides to prevent high blood pressure in the first place. If you have hypertension, you can control it working in partnership with your physician. By preventing or controlling high blood pressure, you can lower your risk of heart disease, kidney failure, stroke, and many other serious conditions associated with the damage it causes to your arteries and organs. An added bonus: You'll benefit from enhanced physical well-being, and you'll probably enjoy life more, too.

Understanding Hypertension: The Silent Killer

Hypertension is called the *silent killer,* because it typically does not cause any noticeable symptoms. The result:

✔ Almost 31 percent of adults in the United States have high blood pressure.

✔ Only 47 percent of adults with high blood pressure have it under control.

- About 1 in 5 people with hypertension don't know it.
- About 7 in 10 people with high blood pressure take medicine to control it. Of these, only 64 percent have their blood pressure effectively controlled.

But you don't have to be part of this trend. You can take simple steps in your daily life to lower your risk of high blood pressure. If you are already at risk or have hypertension, you can work with your physician to control it effectively. It may take some time and adjustment, but you can do it. The place to start is with a little education.

Defining blood pressure

As the heart pumps blood through the circulatory system, the blood that's being pumped exerts pressure against the interior walls of the blood vessels. Your *blood pressure* reading consists of two measurements of the pressure exerted on the walls of the arteries. These measurements are expressed in millimeters (mm) of mercury (Hg), a measure of pressure. For example, 110mm/70 mm Hg (read "one hundred-ten over seventy millimeters of mercury") or 120/80 mm Hg are two typical readings for *normal blood pressure*. The top or higher number is called the *systolic pressure,* which expresses the pressure exerted as the heart contracts or beats, pumping blood through the circulatory system. The bottom, or lower number, is called *diastolic pressure,* which expresses the pressure exerted when the heart is at rest between beats.

Defining high blood pressure

Many people mistakenly think that you either have hypertension or you don't. In fact, blood pressure readings span a continuum ranging all the way from *normal* to *severely elevated.* Experiencing one elevated reading does not mean that you have hypertension. Everyone's blood pressure tends to spike up in situations that produce anger, pain, fear, or high stress. For example, your blood pressure probably rises when you have a shouting match with a family member, give a speech, or interview for a new position — maybe even when you visit your friendly doctor. Blood pressure also varies during the day. It's usually lower when you are resting or sleeping, for example.

Having *hypertension* means that your blood pressure is consistently elevated above the normal ranges. (It doesn't mean that you are supertense. Even the calmest, most laid-back individuals can have high blood pressure.) And knowing whether you have it is no do-it-yourself diagnosis, either. You need to have your blood pressure checked regularly, ideally as part of a regular periodic checkup. If you happen to check your blood pressure at a health fair, for example, and it's elevated, be sure to see your physician. Your physician will take your blood pressure readings on several occasions to determine whether your blood pressure is consistently elevated, and if it is, how severely elevated it is.

Identifying categories of blood pressure

For many years, hypertension typically was defined as readings higher than 140/90 mm Hg (measured in millimeters of mercury). This rather arbitrary cutoff was chosen to define high blood pressure because the risk of cardiovascular complication becomes very significant at this point. By the early 2000s, however, a large body of research enabled medical scientists to determine a range of blood pressure classifications that better express the increasing health risks of increasingly higher blood pressure. You can review these classifications in Table 8-1.

Table 8-1	Classification of Blood Pressure for Adults 18 and Older*		
Category	*Systolic (mm Hg)*		*Diastolic (mm Hg)*
Normal	<120	and	<80
Prehypertension	120–139	or	80–89
Hypertension			
Stage 1	140–159	or	90–99
Stage 2	>160	or	≥100

Key: < less than; > greater than, ≥ or equal to

* Reprinted from The Seventh Report of the Joint National Committee on Prevention, Detection, Evaluation and Treatment of High Blood Pressure. National Institute of Health. National Heart, Lung, and Blood Institute. National High Blood Pressure Education Program. NIH Publication No. 03-5233. May 2003.

Very recently in the U.S., an expert commission recommended modifications of some of these ranges when used as target goals for measuring and controlling high blood pressure in such groups as older adults (those 60 years of age or older) and adults who already have high blood pressure. These recommendations don't change the definition of high blood pressure as beginning at 140/90 mm Hg. And the classifications in the table remain very useful for understanding how the risks of damage from high blood pressure increase incrementally as blood pressure rises.

High blood pressure (hypertension)

As Table 8-1 illustrates, people with a systolic blood pressure greater than 139 mm Hg or a diastolic blood pressure greater than 89 mm Hg are considered to have *hypertension*. Hypertension is then further divided into two stages of increasing severity.

Prehypertensive blood pressure

A number of large observational and clinical studies show that people with blood pressure that is elevated from just slightly above normal to just under Stage 1 hypertension levels have at least twice the risk of developing high blood pressure. In addition, research shows that for people ages 40 to 70, the risk of heart disease doubles for every increment of 20 mm Hg in systolic blood pressure (the upper number) and 10 mm Hg in diastolic blood pressure (the bottom number) that their blood pressure goes above 115/75. As a consequence, the scientists established the classification *prehypertension* to alert individuals to this risk and to raise awareness that most people with prehypertensive blood pressure can improve their blood pressure dramatically with a few simple lifestyle modifications.

Normal blood pressure

The other important category in this classification system is *normal blood pressure*. Individuals with a systolic blood pressure of less than 120 mm Hg and a diastolic blood pressure of less than 80 mm Hg are considered to have normal blood pressure.

This definition of normal lowers the upper limits of normal from older definitions, because maintaining blood pressure below this level presents the lowest risk for developing heart disease, stroke, kidney disease, and other conditions associated with high blood pressure. Another way to describe this category for healthy people without other risk factors for heart disease or other health problems is *optimal* blood pressure.

Low blood pressure

Is it possible to have blood pressure that's too low? Yes. But you have to have a very low blood pressure, indeed, before it becomes a problem, called *hypotension*. People who have systolic blood pressure less than 90 and diastolic pressure of less than 60 (less than 90/60 mm Hg) may have blood pressure that is too low. Individuals with too low blood pressure may feel dizzy periodically, especially when standing up. For the vast majority of people, however, the range of normal blood pressure is so great that *normal* remains an important distinction. Depending upon your individual situation, your physician may advise you that your optimal blood pressure should be well below the upper limits of normal.

Understanding the Dangers and Causes of Hypertension

Hypertension isn't called a killer for nothing. High blood pressure is a significant risk factor for developing coronary heart disease (CHD), the leading cause of death in the United States. It's also a significant risk for stroke, heart failure, and kidney failure. Anyone with poorly treated hypertension at least doubles his or her risk of developing all of these conditions. And remember, the higher the blood pressure, the higher the danger.

Thus, even individuals who have no symptoms when initially diagnosed with hypertension need to work hard to control blood pressure to prevent these potentially devastating complications. When you're already diagnosed with heart disease and hypertension, then controlling your blood pressure within recommended levels is perhaps the most important step you can take toward preventing or slowing the progress of your heart disease.

Determining the causes of hypertension

In the vast majority (more than 90 percent) of people with high blood pressure, physicians aren't able to determine its exact cause. In medical terms, this condition is known as *primary* or *idiopathic* hypertension. That's not to say that physicians are idiots, but that they haven't yet figured out the precise mechanisms, functions, or agents that cause hypertension. Primary hypertension is also termed *essential* high blood pressure. In the same way that *idiopathic* doesn't mean that doctors are idiots, neither does *essential* mean that having hypertension is essential. Quite the contrary! Treating it is what *is* essential! Look at some of the factors that appear to contribute to hypertension.

- **Salt intake:** Among the theories about what causes primary high blood pressure, most relate to problems that your kidneys appear to have with handling excess salt. Population studies show that societies in which people consume large amounts of salt (such as the United States) have a correspondingly high incidence of high blood pressure. Similarly, in cultures where salt intake is low, the incidence of high blood pressure is extremely low. Other studies show that for most people with hypertension, restricting salt intake helps lower high blood pressure.

- **Inherited predisposition:** Hypertension also appears to have a genetic component. Some people may be genetically predisposed to have high blood pressure. However, although hypertension runs in some families, these tendencies may actually result as much from shared lifestyles as they do from shared genetic backgrounds. Doctors certainly know that lifestyle factors, such as obesity (and abdominal obesity, in particular), inactivity, cigarette smoking, and high alcohol consumption all are associated with increased risk of hypertension.

✔ **Known conditions that cause it:** In approximately 10 percent of the people with hypertension, the specific underlying cause can be discovered. This condition is known as *secondary hypertension,* meaning it's a secondary result of a separate primary condition. If the underlying condition can be treated and corrected, then secondary hypertension usually is corrected, too. Conditions known to cause secondary high blood pressure include

- • Narrowing of the arteries that supply the kidneys

- • Other diseases of the kidneys

- • Abnormalities in the endocrine system, such as overactive adrenal glands or a benign tumor in the adrenal glands that secretes a hormone that raises blood pressure.

- • Transient conditions such as pregnancy for certain women

- • Certain medications that can increase the risk of high blood pressure, such as oral contraceptives or estrogen replacement therapy following menopause

If you're diagnosed with high blood pressure, your doctor will explore any of these potential underlying causes for hypertension prior to making the diagnosis.

Checking out other important risk factors

Although medical science may not know the exact mechanisms that cause primary hypertension, a number of conditions are strongly associated with increases in high blood pressure. Arresting any one of this gang of probable causes usually leads to lower blood pressure. For many people, controlling these conditions actually returns their blood pressure to normal levels:

✔ **Obesity:** Hypertension is most clearly associated with obesity (weighing more than 20 percent above your desirable body weight). Obesity contributes to an estimated 40 percent or more of all high blood pressure cases in the United States. Although not everyone who is overweight has high blood pressure, the association remains crystal clear.

✔ **Physical inactivity:** People who are physically inactive increase their likelihood of developing high blood pressure. In one large study of more than 16,000 individuals, inactive people were 35 percent more likely to develop hypertension than were active people, regardless of whether they had a family history of high blood pressure or a personal history of being overweight.

- ✔ **Cigarette smoking:** Cigarette smoking and the use of other tobacco products increase blood pressure, both in the short term while you're smoking or chewing and in the long term, because components in the smoke or chewing tobacco, such as nicotine, cause your arteries to constrict. Childhood experiments with the nozzle on a garden hose indicate what happens when you force the same volume of liquid through a smaller opening. That higher pressure isn't a happy thing for your arteries.

- ✔ **Alcohol intake:** Drinking small to moderate amounts of alcohol (two drinks daily or fewer for men and one drink daily for women) has been shown in a number of studies to reduce mortality from CHD. Higher consumption of alcohol, however, clearly is associated with increased blood pressure, not to mention an increased risk of dying from heart disease.

Looking at hypertension in specific groups of people

Having high blood pressure raises some special issues for certain groups of people.

Children and adolescents

Children and adolescents who have blood pressures at levels in the top 5 percent for their age groups are considered to have elevated blood pressure. Seeking the potential underlying causes is mandatory in all children and adolescents who have high blood pressure. Because children are more likely to have secondary causes for hypertension than are adults, physicians look for conditions such as abnormalities of the aorta or kidney problems that are associated with high blood pressure. Overweight and physical inactivity can also put children at risk.

In most instances, treatment for children and adolescents with elevated blood pressure involves lifestyle measures such as increased physical activity and, if the child is overweight, weight loss. Medicines are used only as a last resort and, even then, usually only for children who have extremely high blood pressure. A child or adolescent with high blood pressure needs to be treated by a pediatric cardiologist or a pediatrician who is knowledgeable in the particular demands of treating high blood pressure in young people.

The elderly

As already indicated, the older you grow, the more likely you are to have high blood pressure. And if you're older than 60 and African American, you have an even greater risk of having hypertension.

Because high blood pressure is so common in older individuals, men and women alike, if you're older than 60, having your blood pressure checked frequently by your physician and paying particular attention to positive lifestyle measures, such as maintenance of normal body weight and regular physical activity, are mandatory.

If you are older, you should also be aware of the risk of a sudden drop in blood pressure that occurs when you stand up. In medical terms, this sudden low blood pressure is called *postural*, or *orthostatic*, hypotension. It often causes dizziness, lightheadedness, and even fainting, which may cause falls. This reaction may result from having heart disease, diabetes, or certain other health conditions, or from taking certain medications, such as some for treating high blood pressure, depression, or Parkinson's disease.

Many individuals purchase one of the automatic blood pressure measuring devices to monitor their blood pressure at home. The most accurate way to measure your own blood pressure with such a device is to read the instructions for use carefully and then use the machine to measure your blood pressure after you have been sitting quietly for several minutes. It is a good idea to write the value you obtain down with the date in order to show it to your doctor at a later date. There is a section about monitoring your own blood pressure later in this chapter.

African Americans

In all age groups (not only those older than 60), adults of African American descent have a higher prevalence of high blood pressure than do Americans of other ethnic groups. Furthermore, the condition appears to be more dangerous in African Americans. Compared with the general U.S. population, African Americans experience 40 percent more high blood pressure, twice the risk of stroke, and six times the rate of hypertension-related kidney failure. African Americans also have been shown to suffer more damage to their kidneys than Caucasians at comparable levels of blood pressure.

Although the causes underlying this difference, like the underlying causes for most hypertension, remain unknown, ongoing research suggests several possibilities.

> ✔ **Later diagnosis and treatment:** Many African Americans may not receive treatment for high blood pressure until they've had the condition for some time and damage to the body has occurred.

✔ **Greater sensitivity to salt:** Recent research suggests that some African Americans have a genetic trait that increases salt sensitivity and its corresponding effect on elevating blood pressure.

✔ **High salt and low potassium intake:** Many African Americans eat diets that are high in salt and low in potassium, both factors associated with elevated blood pressure.

Fortunately, research shows that when African Americans receive appropriate treatment using current therapies, their success in controlling blood pressure equals that of Caucasians and other ethnic groups receiving equivalent treatment. Because of the prevalence of high blood pressure and earlier onset, if you're an African American, you need to be sure to have your blood pressure checked regularly, and the childhood or teenage years are not too early.

People with diabetes mellitus

High blood pressure is much more common in individuals with diabetes than it is in the general population; moreover, it is particularly dangerous for them, because it carries a high risk of cardiovascular complications. Individuals with high blood pressure *and* diabetes are extremely susceptible to this *double trouble,* because of the increased risk of suffering damage to their kidneys, which, in turn, increases the risk of high blood pressure. For all these reasons, individuals with diabetes need to be carefully monitored for high blood pressure, and this condition needs to be treated aggressively. Consult with your doctor for the treatment that is right for you.

Pregnancy

Some women develop high blood pressure during the third trimester of pregnancy. This condition is called *gestational hypertension,* and it needs to be treated cautiously by a physician who is familiar with the patient and this condition. The physician must also carefully distinguish gestational hypertension from *preeclampsia,* which is a potentially lethal condition. Fortunately, women who develop gestational hypertension have no apparent increased risk of hypertension following the pregnancy, compared with the general population.

If a pregnant woman has been diagnosed with hypertension before she becomes pregnant, or if she develops it before the 20th week of pregnancy, she is described as having *chronic hypertension.* This condition also needs to be treated by a physician experienced with treating high blood pressure during pregnancy.

The goal of treating high blood pressure during pregnancy, regardless of whether it's gestational or chronic, is lowering any health risks to the pregnant woman and the baby. For these reasons, and many others, prenatal care is important for all pregnant women.

Taking Charge of Your Blood Pressure

Controlling many of your daily habits and practices can help you prevent high blood pressure or manage existing hypertension. Taking these lifestyle measures also is an important part of treatment even if you require medicines to control your blood pressure.

Managing your weight

For overweight individuals, even those who are only 15 or 20 pounds overweight, weight reduction is a highly reliable way of lowering blood pressure.

Most studies indicate that you lose approximately 1 mm Hg from both your systolic and diastolic blood pressure for every two pounds that you lose. Thus, even small amounts of weight loss can make a profound difference in blood-pressure control. Many individuals who lose 10 to 15 pounds can anticipate a 5 mm Hg to 7 mm Hg reduction in their systolic and diastolic blood pressure levels. For that reason, your doctor is likely to first recommend weight reduction if you're overweight and have high blood pressure. If you are overweight but do not have elevated blood pressure, losing weight is a frontline strategy to prevent getting it. See Chapter 10 for programs for effective weight loss.

Getting regular physical activity

Use it (your body) and lose it (your high blood pressure). Physically active individuals reduce their risk of developing hypertension by 20 percent to 50 percent when compared with their couch potato peers. So getting 30 to 45 minutes of moderate-intensity exercise on most days of the week helps keep your blood pressure normal. This is true even for many older adults.

Individuals who already have hypertension can often lower their systolic blood pressure by 5 mm Hg to10 mm Hg simply by participating in moderately intense aerobic activity 30 to 45 minutes most days of the week. If you have hypertension, you

✔ Must conduct your physical activity at a *moderate level,* which means reducing the intensity of your exercise to a level slightly less than that recommended for individuals your age without hypertension (see Chapter 5 for more details about moderate exercise).

✔ Don't need to take your 30 to 45 minutes of physical activity all at one time but may accumulate it during the course of the day.

The benefits of regular physical activity for controlling blood pressure are added to those of weight loss.

Eating a low-sodium, heart-healthy diet

Many aspects of proper nutrition play significant roles in blood pressure control, so adopting a heart-healthy way of eating is a wise choice (see Chapter 5). A heart-healthy diet emphasizes vegetables, fruits, legumes, whole grains, low-fat dairy and healthy oils while limiting saturated fats and eliminating trans fats.

Perhaps most important, however, individuals with high blood pressure need to consume a diet that is low in sodium. The American Heart Association recommends that everyone eat a diet that contains no more than 2,300 milligrams of sodium a day. That's equivalent to about 1 teaspoon of table salt. The recommended daily limit is 1,500 milligrams (about ¾ teaspoon) for people over 50 and for those who have heart disease, diabetes, high blood pressure, and other health conditions.

The best ways to lower sodium in your diet are by

- ✔ Removing the saltshaker from the table
- ✔ Not adding extra salt to food
- ✔ Emphasizing fresh fruits and vegetables and whole grains
- ✔ Avoiding salty snacks and processed foods

Your doctor, often working in conjunction with a registered dietitian, can help you build a plan for eating that achieves these goals. This plan may include a role for increasing potassium in your diet. Fresh fruits and vegetables often are often high in potassium.

Avoiding tobacco use

Cigarette smoking, chewing tobacco, and other uses of tobacco have been repeatedly shown to raise blood pressure. The good news is that within a few months after quitting cigarette smoking, you'll experience a significant reduction in your blood pressure. I discuss the benefits of quitting in Chapter 11.

Limiting alcohol intake

If you consume alcoholic beverages, do so only in moderation (no more than two alcoholic drinks a day if you're a man and one if you're a woman). If having a few drinks with friends is the way you unwind at the end of the day, try some alternative ways of relaxing — join a gym or aerobics class, check out the local coffee (decaffeinated, of course) shops, or play a team sport.

Chilling out to reduce stress

If you're in a stressful environment, finding ways to reduce stress often helps lower your blood pressure. Check out the suggestions in Chapter 6.

Working with Your Doctor to Control Your Blood Pressure

If you want to succeed in combating high blood pressure, which has no imme-diate symptoms and lasts for many years, you need to develop a long-term partnership with your physician. Doing so typically involves three stages.

Getting a medical evaluation

The diagnosis of high blood pressure requires at least two or three different blood pressure readings on separate visits to your doctor's office, indicating that your blood pressure is consistently greater than 140/90 mm Hg.

If your blood pressure is elevated above 120/80 mm Hg to just under 140/90 mm Hg, you may have prehypertensive blood pressure (see the earlier section "Prehypertensive blood pressure"). In that case, your doctor may ask you to help in the diagnosis by monitoring your blood pressure at home. A number of excellent home monitoring devices are available that can provide accurate readings at home, and your doctor may recommend one.

 Don't be surprised if your blood pressure is slightly lower at home than it is at the doctor's office. This phenomenon is called the *white coat syndrome,* because a number of people get nervous in their doctor's office, and being nervous is one of the emotional states that can elevate blood pressure temporarily.

Determining treatment

The second phase in combating hypertension is treatment. Depending upon the severity of your hypertension, your physician may first ask you to make some of the lifestyle changes I discuss earlier in this chapter to help control your blood pressure. Your doctor may also prescribe medications in con-junction with these lifestyle measures to provide additional blood pressure control. I discuss more about medications in the "Using medicines to treat hypertension" section later in this chapter.

Self-monitoring

After diagnosing your high blood pressure, your doctor normally asks you to participate as a partner in your own care by

✔ Monitoring and keeping a log of your blood pressure.

✔ Following prescribed lifestyle modifications with commitment.

✔ Taking your medication (if it's prescribed) faithfully and as directed.

Astonishingly, more than 50 percent of all medicines prescribed either are not taken at all or not taken correctly. Controlling your blood pressure is virtually impossible if you don't meticulously follow prescribed lifestyle measures and medication regimens.

✔ Honestly sharing with your doctor any problems or side effects you're having with either lifestyle modifications or medications. Doing so often is a crucial key to your success, because it enables you and your doctor to make necessary adjustments.

Don't worry that you'll be a bother — doctors know that it can take time to fine-tune a treatment regimen to work best for you. If your doctor seems too rushed or reluctant to work with you, find one who isn't.

Selecting a home blood pressure monitor

Many brands and types of home blood pressure monitors are available. Either of the following basic types may work well for you. If you're not sure how to operate the device you select, the staff in your doctor's office will be happy to show you. For all monitors, you must have a cuff that fits your arm; if you have a larger arm, too small a cuff can lead to inaccurate measurements.

✔ **Electronic or digital monitor:** Advances in the sensitivity and reliability of electronic monitoring devices have made these monitors reliably accurate when used as directed. Because they're easy to use, have clear displays, work with one hand, and don't require the use of a stethoscope, many people prefer them. They come in versions that have either manually or automatically inflated cuffs. Reliable digital wrist monitors also are available.

Warning: Avoid small digital finger monitors and the like (often sold in cheap mail-order catalogs), because most of these so-called monitors are highly inaccurate and a waste of your money.

✔ **Aneroid monitors:** These monitors have a dial gauge, cuff, inflator bulb, and stethoscope. If you choose one of these, you may want to make sure that the cuff has a D-ring for easy one-handed use and a self-bleeding deflation valve so that you can concentrate on measuring accurately (rather than on trying to let the air out properly).

Whatever monitor you select, be sure that you follow the manufacturer's instructions to the letter. Remember, if you need help, ask your doctor's staff for some basic instruction.

Using medicines to treat hypertension

To medicate or not to medicate? That is the question. When Hamlet raised his famous question, "To be or not to be," he was voicing a philosophical dilemma. Your physician often faces the dilemma of whether you need medication in addition to lifestyle measures. Medicines are definitely indicated whenever positive lifestyle measures haven't succeeded in adequately lowering your blood pressure. In this situation, your physician has many excellent medications to choose from.

Adding to the dilemma, different medications also work differently for different individuals. So a period of adjustment may be needed to find out just which medication or combination of medications works best for you. Treatment guidelines note that most individuals require two or more medications used simultaneously to reach blood pressure goals. If your doctor needs to combine several medications, they often will come from different classes.

The following three general classes of medications typically are used in controlling high blood pressure.

- ✔ **Diuretics:** The first choice of many physicians, diuretics lower blood pressure by lowering blood volume through increasing the amount of sodium and water passed through the kidneys. With regular diuretic therapy, blood pressure often falls 10 mm Hg.

- ✔ **Alpha blockers and beta blockers:** These medications inhibit various portions of the nervous system, particularly receptors called *alpha* and *beta receptors*. Inhibiting them helps lower blood pressure by slowing the heart rate and decreasing the force with which the heart pumps or by helping arteries to relax or dilate, thus lowering the pressure required to pump blood through the arteries.

- ✔ **Vasodilators:** These drugs act directly on the walls of the arteries and cause them to relax, thereby reducing the amount of pressure needed to pump blood through the arteries. The major types of vasodilators in use are

  - • **ACE inhibitors:** These drugs help reduce blood pressure by decreasing substances in the blood that cause vessels to constrict. The acronym ACE stands for *angiotensin converting enzyme*. Both short-acting (taken several times a day) and long-acting (typically taken once a day) ACE inhibitors are available for treatment of high blood pressure. Your physician may want to monitor kidney function and potassium levels closely when starting or increasing this medication.

- **Angiotensin II receptor blockers (ARBs):** ARBs block the action, rather than the creation, of chemicals that narrow the blood vessels. They may work better than ACE inhibitors for some people.

- **Calcium antagonists:** Also called *calcium channel blockers,* calcium antagonists inhibit the inward flow of calcium into cardiac and blood vessel tissues, thereby reducing the tension of the heart and the constriction of blood vessels.

✔ **Combination medicines:** As I mention in the previous section, the majority of people require two medicines to control their high blood pressure. Obtaining those medications in a combined form often is possible and makes taking them simpler. If you're taking two or more medications for hypertension, ask your doctor whether a combination medicine is right for you.

Ten tips for controlling your blood pressure for a lifetime

Because complications from high blood pressure are the result of years of increased pressure pounding on blood vessels walls, adopting a lifelong approach to controlling hypertension is important. Remember that the goal is not simply to lower blood pressure in the short term but rather to reduce the long-term devastating complications of hypertension.

To achieve that goal, follow these ten tips:

✔ Become knowledgeable about hypertension.

✔ Make a commitment to help your physician control your blood pressure by actively joining in a partnership to assist in your therapy.

✔ Maintain regular contact with your physician.

✔ Adopt a heart-healthy diet, such as the DASH diet or the Mediterranean diet, that helps to lower blood pressure.

✔ Get 30 to 45 minutes of moderate intensity exercise on most days of the week.

✔ Routinely monitor your blood pressure at home.

✔ Take your medicines the way your doctor prescribes them.

✔ Integrate medicine-taking into your daily living routines.

✔ Monitor side effects and report any troublesome ones to your physician.

✔ Maintain a positive attitude about achieving the goal of life-long blood pressure control.

Treating resistant hypertension

Some individuals have a condition called *resistant hypertension*. These individuals often require a combination of lifestyle measures coupled with two or three medications to control their high blood pressure. If you experience this situation, keep working closely with your physician.

Blood pressure can almost always be controlled, even if you have resistant hypertension, provided that you meticulously follow the regimens that are developed in partnership with your physician.

Chapter 9

Managing Bad (and Good) Cholesterol

In This Chapter

▶ Understanding how elevated cholesterol multiplies your risk of coronary heart disease

▶ Finding out about lipids — cholesterol, lipoproteins, and triglycerides

▶ Lowering your cholesterol using lifestyle measures or medications

▶ Controlling deadly duos — cholesterol and hypertension, and cholesterol and diabetes

Cholesterol always seems to be in the news. For a while, Americans were so obsessed with lowering blood cholesterol that other important risk factors for heart disease were almost ignored. Then the pendulum swung the other way as revisionists began underestimating the dangers of elevated cholesterol levels. The truth lies somewhere in between.

Without question, elevated blood cholesterol significantly increases — doubles, in fact — the risk of developing coronary heart disease (CHD). And in combination with other risk factors, such as high blood pressure, overweight, or obesity, cholesterol multiplies those risks many times over. So controlling cholesterol is vital to lowering your risk of developing heart disease and to controlling the progression of heart disease if you have it.

For most people, achieving that goal usually isn't hard: Some simple daily steps can make a great difference. Eating a heart-healthy diet, getting regular physical activity, and keeping weight in the normal range enables most people to keep their cholesterol levels low risk. Even if you have cholesterol problems (dyslipidemia) or heart disease and must take medication to control these issues, lifestyle steps form the foundation of therapy.

Hearing the Good News/Bad News about Cholesterol

The good news is that between the 1960s and the late 2000s, the average total cholesterol level in the United States decreased from 220 mg/dL (milligrams per deciliter) to about 200 mg/dL. This drop no doubt contributed to a 50 percent decline during the past 30 years in the incidence of death from heart disease. The bad news is that elevated blood cholesterol remains extremely common, and heart disease still is the leading killer in the U.S. An estimated 32 percent of American adults have elevated blood cholesterol levels or other lipid issues that put them at increased risk for developing heart disease.

The risk of elevated total cholesterol and LDL cholesterol (the "bad" cholesterol) increases as you age. Factors such as gender, genetics, and ethnicity also affect cholesterol levels. So being aware of how cholesterol affects heart health is a smart idea.

The relationship between cholesterol levels and the risk of developing heart disease doesn't function like a light bulb — meaning that it's either on or off. It's more like the gradual acceleration your car experiences entering a freeway. As cholesterol in the blood gradually rises to a level of about 200 mg/dL and LDL tops 100 mg/dL, the risk of developing heart disease also gradually increases. After your cholesterol goes above those levels, the risk of heart disease and of dying from heart disease increases much more rapidly. By the time your cholesterol level reaches 250, your risk of dying from heart disease grows to more than twice that of individuals whose cholesterol levels are below 200.

But good news! The reverse also is true. Lowering your blood cholesterol level by even a smidgen can make a positive difference. And the more you lower it, the greater the benefit. For every one point that your cholesterol drops, estimates indicate your risk of heart disease drops by 2 percent. Thus, a drop of 10 mg/dL in your cholesterol level can decrease your risk of developing heart disease by 20 percent! (Wouldn't you love returns like that on your IRA?)

Getting the Lowdown on Lipids

The term *lipids* in medicine describes fats. There now, don't you know a lot more? Would it help if I told you that *lipid* comes from the Greek word for *fat?* (Yes, *fat* as in *lipo*suction.) In the body, lipids play an important part in cell structure and serve as fuel. They are easily stored. Lipids of most concern in heart disease include cholesterol, low-density lipoprotein cholesterol (LDL-C), high-density lipoprotein cholesterol (HDL-C), and triglycerides.

Comprehending cholesterol

Cholesterol is a naturally occurring waxy substance present in human beings and all other animals. It is an important component of the body's cell walls. The body also requires cholesterol to produce many hormones (including sex hormones) and the bile acids that help it digest food. Because cholesterol plays such important biological roles, having adequate amounts of it is absolutely essential for life itself.

Humans get cholesterol mainly from two sources. The liver manufactures a great deal, and you consume some from animal products, such as meat, eggs, and dairy products. However, you get into trouble when you have too much cholesterol, particularly LDL cholesterol, in your blood. Your level of blood cholesterol (sometimes called *serum cholesterol*) grows too high usually because you eat too much saturated fat, trans fat, or very refined, simple carbohydrates (which encourage the liver to manufacture cholesterol) and too many foods that contain cholesterol (dietary cholesterol).

Actually, you don't need to consume foods with cholesterol because your body always makes enough. In fact, in years of research, no one has ever been diagnosed with a cholesterol deficiency.

To get to where it needs to go in your body, cholesterol is carried around in your bloodstream, attached to complicated structures called *lipoproteins*. When cholesterol levels in the blood are too high, excess lipids are deposited on the inside walls of the arteries in the form of *plaque,* which causes arteries to narrow. The result is the condition known as *atherosclerosis,* which is the basis of CHD, as I explain in Chapter 2.

These deposits of lipids cause irritation (known medically as inflammation) that leads to an attempted healing process. Unfortunately, the healing process in this case just makes things worse, eventually causing scarring and calcium formation in the artery wall. The scarring and calcium formation narrow the channel of the artery and hinder the normal flow of blood needed to nourish the cells of the body. Refer to Chapter 2 for details on this process.

Understanding lipoproteins: The good, the bad, and the ugly

A *lipoprotein* is a cross between a lipid, such as cholesterol or triglycerides, and a protein. Because fats and water don't mix well, lipoprotein serves as the mode of transportation for cholesterol and other lipids through the bloodstream, which is mostly water. Lipoproteins are sort of like a cruise ship steaming across the Atlantic Ocean. View the ship as the proteins, and all the passengers on board (including the Family Cholesterol) as the lipids. Not a perfect analogy, but you get the point.

Lipoproteins can be separated and measured according to their weight and density. They range from very low density to high density. They also range in size from small to large. Lipoproteins also have many different constituent proteins called *apoproteins* (*apo*, for short). But you need not get that deep into biochemistry to understand how two types of lipoprotein function in creating or fighting atherosclerosis.

One particularly dangerous form is called LDL or *low-density lipoprotein. LDL* is dangerous, because it contains more fat and less protein and easily adheres to artery walls, particularly where they are damaged, and enters into plaque formation. Because LDL cholesterol plays such a major role in forming atherosclerotic plaque, lowering LDL levels in the blood is an important goal in controlling cholesterol.

On the other hand, a beneficial type of lipoprotein called *HDL,* or *high-density lipoprotein,* can actually help protect your heart from heart disease. HDL doesn't adhere to artery walls. Instead, it actually helps carry cholesterol away from artery walls. This effect is particularly important for the coronary arteries. Research also suggests that HDL is an antioxidant and anti-inflammatory regulator that prevents oxidation of LDL and helps block its plaque-forming properties. Thus, keeping HDL at recommended levels helps control overall cholesterol and its potential negative effects.

When you have a checkup, your doctor may look at the results of your blood tests and say, "Well, you need to work on raising your *good cholesterol* and lowering your *bad cholesterol."* That can be a little confusing until you realize that their names offer you a tip for keeping track of which is which. You want to keep your high-density lipoproteins (HDLs) *high* and your low-density lipoproteins (LDLs) *low.* Repeat after me: High, *high!* Low, *low!* Forgetting this mantra can result in ugly consequences for your arteries.

Tracking elevated blood triglycerides

Fats also are carried through the bloodstream in a form known as triglycerides. Although *triglycerides,* like cholesterol, are lipids, they have a different makeup. As the name suggests, these chemicals are made up of three (hence *tri*) fat molecules (fatty acids) carried through the bloodstream on a glycerol backbone. Much like cholesterol, the triglycerides are ferried around the bloodstream by joining with proteins in the form of lipoproteins. Although the link between elevated blood triglycerides and heart disease isn't as strong as the link between LDL cholesterol and heart disease, having elevated blood triglycerides nevertheless puts you at increased risk for CHD. So to help prevent or reverse atherosclerosis, you also want to keep triglycerides within recommended levels.

Testing Your Cholesterol and Other Lipid Levels

Lowering total cholesterol and LDL cholesterol to desirable levels and raising HDL cholesterol above low levels can slow down, stop, or even reverse the buildup of harmful plaque in your arteries, thus lowering your risk of developing heart disease and experiencing a heart attack. If you want to control this risk fact, knowing your "numbers" is the place to start.

Therefore, in your battle to lower cholesterol, to be at your best, you have to test. It's as simple as that. All adults (and most children) should know their respective cholesterol levels. A simple finger-stick blood test is all that's required for testing total cholesterol. You should have such a test at least every five years, or more often if your cholesterol level is elevated or if you have other risk factors for heart disease.

If the simple test shows your cholesterol level is elevated, your physician may recommend that you undergo a fasting blood test called a complete *lipid profile* or *lipid analysis* to determine your levels of LDL, HDL, and triglycerides. Physicians often include this more extensive test as part of your routine physical checkup.

If you take a simple test outside your doctor's office, perhaps at a health fair, and your cholesterol level measures 200 mg/dL or higher, be sure that you share this information with your physician so you get proper follow-up.

Decoding your cholesterol test results

Your overall cholesterol level is expressed as a number of milligrams (mg) per deciliter (dL — 1/10 of a liter) of blood: 200 mg/dL or 220 mg/dL, for example. A fasting blood test to obtain a complete lipid profile also expresses the levels of LDL and HDL as milligrams per deciliter (mg/dL). The results may also compare the level of HDL (the good guys, remember) to your total cholesterol level. This comparison is usually expressed as a ratio; for example, 3:1 or 4.5:1 means that you have one unit of HDL for every 3 or 4.5 equal units of total cholesterol. (Sometimes just the first number appears on the test report; the 1 is implied.) The most exciting thing about this arcane knowledge, however, is that you don't need even the foggiest idea of what milligrams or deciliters are to understand how to use these numbers effectively.

Equating cholesterol levels with risk of heart disease

Analysis of a large body of research has informed general cholesterol guidelines that are widely used by physicians and medical research scientists in detecting, evaluating, and treating cholesterol problems.

Here are some general guidelines for interpreting what your cholesterol measurements indicate about your risk of developing heart disease or of experiencing increased complications if you already have it:

- ✔ **"Desirable" cholesterol level — 200 mg/dL and lower.** If you don't already have existing CHD, a total cholesterol level below 200 mg/dL is considered a *desirable blood cholesterol*. But please remember that within a broad range of values, lower is better. Thus, a cholesterol level of 170 mg/dL is better than a cholesterol level of 190 mg/dL.

- ✔ **Borderline high blood cholesterol — 200 mg/dL to 239 mg/dL.** If your cholesterol is within this range, your physician will strongly recommend lifestyle modifications and perhaps medication depending on your current practices and risk factors.

- ✔ **High blood cholesterol level — 240 mg/dL or greater.** This classification puts you at high risk. Your physician typically will work closely with you to establish an aggressive treatment program that will likely include lifestyle changes and medication.

In recent years, extensive research, particularly clinical trials, has identified LDL cholesterol as perhaps the lipid of most concern in the development of atherosclerosis. As a result, lowering LDL has also become a primary target for preventing atherosclerosis in the first place and controlling (or even reversing) the process after it results in CHD and other manifestations of heart disease. In fact, new guidelines from the American Heart Association and American College of Cardiology recommend (in addition to lifestyle therapies) more aggressive treatment with statin medications of certain groups of people:

- ✔ **Optimal LDL Cholesterol Level — 100 mg/dL and lower.** If your LDL cholesterol levels are optimal and you have no other risk factors for heart disease (such as high blood pressure, diabetes, or overweight), most physicians will recommend using lifestyle measures that keep your LDL as low as possible. It's never too early to pay attention to these bad actors.

- ✔ **At Risk LDL Cholesterol Levels — 100 mg/dL and above.** Although a LDL of 100 to 129 mg/dL has been consider just above optimal, new treatment guidelines urge physicians to begin targeting LDL more aggressively, using lifestyle measures and appropriate statin or other medication. So be sure to talk to your doctor about what is right for you. Certainly, LDL levels above 130 mg/dL need lowering.

✔ **Low HDL Cholesterol Levels — 40 mg/dL and lower.** A low HDL cholesterol level also is considered an independent risk factor for heart disease, over and above total cholesterol and LDL levels. Individuals whose HDL is below 40 mg/dL should take steps to raise it, usually to close to 60 mg/dL.

✔ **Triglycerides.** If your triglycerides are below 129 mg/dL, they're considered to be *optimal or near optimal.* This recommended classification, may be much lower than you are aware. It takes into account the associations between triglycerides and other lipid and nonlipid risk factors. In addition to increasing your risk of CHD, very high levels of triglycerides may also injure the pancreas, a vital organ that is responsible for producing insulin in the body.

Treating and Managing Cholesterol Problems

Here's a riddle for you: How is cholesterol control different from spandex? When it comes to controlling cholesterol, one size definitely doesn't fit all. In determining how best to control your cholesterol, your physician takes into account not only your cholesterol level and personal history but also a number of other factors, such as your age and gender and whether you already have CHD. The intensity and components of a plan vary depending on these factors, but in all cases, treatment focuses on positive lifestyle factors, such as proper nutrition, increased physical activity, and optimal weight management.

Taking an overview of typical cholesterol treatment

By first looking at an overview of how cholesterol usually is controlled you can then find out more about some specific individual situations. Here are typical treatments for various cholesterol levels:

✔ **If your cholesterol level is at or below 200 mg/dL and you show neither evidence of CHD nor other major risk factors,** then no treatment is necessary. Just keep eating sensibly and staying active.

✔ **If your cholesterol is elevated (higher than 200 mg/dL) and you have other risk factors, including elevated LDL cholesterol and/or low HDL cholesterol,** then you may undergo a moderately intensive treatment program that focuses on positive lifestyle changes, such as proper nutrition, weight management, and increased physical activities. Your physician may also prescribe medication.

✔ **If your cholesterol is elevated (higher than 200 mg/dL), your LDL is high, or you already have established CHD and/or are at high risk to suffer from its complications such as angina or heart attack,** then you may receive the most intensive therapy, which usually will include substantial lifestyle modifications and medication.

Individualizing cholesterol treatment plans

Now that you're aware of how cholesterol levels usually are controlled, here are some of the treatment plans that focus more on the individual:

✔ **If you have risk factors other than elevated cholesterol,** the approach that you and your physician take to help you manage elevated blood cholesterol should take into account not only your cholesterol and lipid levels but also the other risk factors you exhibit (see Chapter 3). Some risk factors such as hypertension, high LDL, low HDL, and diabetes influence therapies for elevated blood cholesterol.

✔ **If you already have CHD, diabetes, or peripheral vascular disease and may have even suffered a complication, such as angina or heart attack** (see also Chapter 2), the goal of treatment is preventing further complications. In medicine, this technique is known as *secondary prevention* and indicates that the goal is preventing second and third events, or complications, in people who already have an established problem. If you fall into this category, your physician may want to dramatically lower your LDL cholesterol. Many studies show that doing so may reduce the likelihood of further complications of heart disease and may even contribute to reversing heart disease.

✔ **If you have low HDL cholesterol,** remember that you're running an independent increased risk of heart disease, over and above high levels of LDL or total cholesterol. Although not many therapeutic options are available for raising HDL, your physician may certainly recommend that you increase your physical activity, which can help raise HDL. Certain lipid-lowering medications, in particular fibric acids and niacin, also are known for raising HDL levels.

✔ **If you're a young adult, premenopausal woman, or man younger than 35,** your long-term risk of CHD increases if you have an elevated cholesterol level, but you're still considered at moderately low risk. Thus, if you exhibit no other risk factors for heart disease, your physician may recommend improved nutritional practices and weight management (if you're overweight) coupled with increased physical activity (if you're currently sedentary). Medications to lower your cholesterol may be recommended only when your total cholesterol or LDL levels are very high or if you experience other significant risk factors for CHD.

✔ **If you're older,** remember that age is an independent risk factor for heart disease. The older you get, the greater your risk for developing CHD. But if you reach the age of 65, your chance of reaching the age of 80 is greater than 80 percent! Thus, prevention is important — and possible — at any age. Because many older individuals with elevated cholesterol also have other chronic illnesses, seeking the advice of your physician is particularly important, because in this situation, some of the medications for lowering cholesterol interact with medications you're taking for other chronic or acute conditions.

✔ **If you're a woman,** you may underestimate the dangers of CHD — the way all too many women do — and therefore tend to underestimate the importance of controlling cholesterol. Remember that heart disease is the leading cause of death in women as well as in men. This factor is particularly true for postmenopausal women. Blood cholesterol levels among American women increase sharply around age 40 and continue to rising until more than half of women older than 55 need to lower their cholesterol levels.

Managing your cholesterol with three key lifestyle steps

How you choose to conduct your daily life in three important areas can help lower your elevated blood cholesterol. The key lifestyle decisions involve committing yourself to proper nutrition, including low saturated fat and low cholesterol consumption, increasing physical activity, and maintaining a healthy weight.

Eating a heart-smart diet

The overall goals of providing proper nutrition to people with elevated blood cholesterol are to help them lower their cholesterol levels while maintaining a balanced and nutritionally adequate eating pattern. Guidelines for accomplishing these goals emphasize eating a balanced diet of nutrient-dense whole foods (not empty calories) that promote general health as well as heart health and that lower cholesterol. Such eating patterns feature the following:

✔ Vegetables, beans, fruits, and whole-grain foods, which are rich in vitamins, minerals, antioxidants, complex carbohydrates, and dietary fiber

✔ Lean protein such as fish, tofu, poultry, and lower fat cuts of meat

✔ Low-fat dairy

✔ The right balance of fats: more healthful polyunsaturated and monounsaturated fats, limited saturated fats, and no trans fats.

✔ Limited foods with cholesterol such as eggs, whole milk, and higher fat cuts of meat.

✔ Limited refined, simple carbohydrate foods such as refined flours and grains, added sugars. A number of eating plans can adapt to this heart-healthy pattern, including the Mediterranean diet, the DASH diet (developed to help lower blood pressure), and vegetarian or plant-based eating patterns. Check out more dietary specifics in Chapter 5.

Many people suffer from the misconception that food cannot be enjoyable and tasty as part of an eating plan to lower cholesterol (or control high blood pressure). Most of the recipes in this book are compatible with an eating pattern designed to lower cholesterol and are delicious. For an entire book full of such tasty, heart-healthy recipes see *The Healthy Heart Cookbook For Dummies* (John Wiley & Sons, Inc.).

Getting at least 30 minutes of physical activity daily

A sedentary lifestyle, which I discuss at length in Chapter 3, is a strong and established risk factor for CHD. The good news is that increased physical activity — at least 30 minutes a day — not only lowers your overall risk for CHD, but it also helps you with cholesterol problems. Regular aerobic activity actually increases HDL cholesterol, which, in turn, is associated with decreased risk of heart disease. Even moderately intense physical activity, such as brisk walking, can raise HDL cholesterol. Strength training has a role to play also, in part because it builds more muscle, which boosts metabolism and helps manage weight.

Of course, if you've been sedentary or already have established CHD, you need to check with your physician before starting a program of increased physical activity.

Maintaining a healthy weight

Next to proper nutritional practices, weight loss is the most important lifestyle intervention for lowering elevated cholesterol if you're overweight. Weight reduction helps lower your LDL cholesterol, lower triglycerides, and raise HDL cholesterol. People usually underestimate the benefit of weight reduction for correcting lipid problems. Even being 15 or 20 pounds over your optimal weight can contribute to elevated cholesterol levels.

Using drug treatment for high cholesterol

In some instances, managing high cholesterol requires lipid-lowering medications in addition to lifestyle measures. This requirement is of particular necessity if

✔ Your blood cholesterol is extremely high and/or your LDL cholesterol is elevated

✔ You experience other major risk factors for heart disease

✔ You already have established CHD

In these instances, your physician probably will recommend drug therapy, in addition to lifestyle measures, to lower elevated blood cholesterol.

Classifying medications used to treat high cholesterol

Although a bewildering variety of cholesterol medications are available, the major ones fall into one of these categories:

✔ **Statins:** Numerous statin medications help lower blood cholesterol. All of them act on an enzyme that is essential for the body to produce cholesterol. The statins slow down, or inhibit, this enzyme, which is called *HMG-CoA reductase.* (Remember that tongue twister, and you'll probably be one up on your doctor!) Many studies show that these medications powerfully reduce cholesterol and lower the risk of CHD. Statin medicines are particularly useful in lowering high levels of LDL cholesterol. Guidelines recommend them as first-line therapy for most people.

✔ **Bile acid sequestrants:** Also called *bile acid resins,* these medications lower blood cholesterol by first binding with cholesterol-containing bile acids in the intestines. Thus bound together, the bile acids and cholesterol are carried from the body in the stool. Bile acid sequestrants have a long history of safe and effective use for lowering blood cholesterol. However, some side effects, such as indigestion and gas, are more common with bile acid sequestrants than with statins. These medications are particularly valuable if you have elevated LDL cholesterol.

✔ **Fibric acids:** Fibric acids are particularly effective in lowering triglycerides, and they've demonstrated the ability to modestly lower LDL cholesterol. Fibric acids are particularly appropriate if you have high triglyceride levels and elevated LDL cholesterol. Tests also show that some of these medications raise HDL cholesterol — the good guys.

✔ **Nicotinic acid:** Nicotinic acid, which is a form of the B vitamin called niacin, is effective in lowering triglycerides and total blood cholesterol and in raising HDL cholesterol. Despite these benefits, some people may have difficulty tolerating this medication because of its side effects, which include itching and flushing of the skin and gastrointestinal distress.

Although niacin is inexpensive and available over the counter, never self-medicate for cholesterol control, because a physician must monitor you for major dangerous side effects.

Considering the risks of estrogen replacement therapy as cholesterol therapy

Although numerous studies through the years showed that estrogen may lower LDL cholesterol and raise HDL cholesterol, research indicates that starting estrogen replacement therapy (ERT) isn't advisable for women with established CHD. In addition, the estrogen-plus-progestin part of the Women's Health Initiative (WHI) study, which was designed to examine the effectiveness of this type of hormone replacement therapy in preventing CHD in postmenopausal women who did not have it, was terminated early because health risks outweighed the benefits. Because other clinically proven medications and therapies effectively lower cholesterol (and treat osteoporosis — another potential benefit of ERT), a number of health organizations now recommend ERT only for short-term relief of the symptoms of menopause. Because of the continuing controversy surrounding ERT, fully discussing of the pros and cons of this approach for treating menopause symptoms with your physician is essential.

Following up after beginning drug therapy

If your physician starts you on medication to help lower cholesterol, having your cholesterol level tested in four to six weeks after beginning the therapy is important. If adequate blood cholesterol lowering isn't achieved, increasing the dosage or adding a second medication may be necessary. Remember, lipid-lowering medications should always be used in conjunction with positive lifestyle measures, such as proper nutrition, increased physical activity, and weight management, if you're overweight.

Regarding Special Issues in Controlling Cholesterol

Addressing special issues is an important part of you and your physician working together to lower blood cholesterol. Other health conditions you may have can influence the therapies your doctor recommends for lowering your cholesterol.

Lowering triglyceride levels

Many steps that you take in your daily life can effectively help lower blood triglycerides, including increasing your physical activity, reducing your weight if you're overweight, and restricting alcohol, simple sugars, and refined or simple carbohydrates in the diet. (Is this beginning to sound familiar?) If your triglyceride levels are elevated in addition to cholesterol, various medications, in particular the fibric acids and nicotinic acid may be added to lifestyle measures to help control high triglycerides and high LDL. Research continues in this area, so be sure to discuss triglyceride control with your doctor.

Delivering a double whammy — high blood cholesterol and hypertension

Elevated blood cholesterol and elevated blood pressure (hypertension) are common afflictions in the U.S. Unfortunately, they frequently occur in tandem, and that spells double trouble because risk factors for heart disease do not add up — they multiply. For example, having elevated blood cholesterol and hypertension quadruples your risk of developing heart disease. Unfortunately, high cholesterol and high blood pressure occur together in 40 percent to 50 percent of people who initially were diagnosed with one or the other condition. This deadly combination is particularly common in overweight individuals.

If you have elevated cholesterol and high blood pressure, you must work with your physician to simultaneously lower both conditions. Controlling the combination of high blood pressure and elevated cholesterol represents a real challenge, because some of the medications used to treat one of the problems may react negatively with the other. Once again, the first line of treatment if you're overweight is weight reduction. Other lifestyle measures, such as proper nutrition and increased physical activity, can simultaneously lower elevated blood pressure and blood cholesterol. (For more information about treating hypertension, see Chapter 8.)

Multiplying trouble — elevated blood cholesterol accompanied by diabetes

Besides hypertension, another dangerous condition frequently associated with elevated blood cholesterol is type 2 diabetes. The lipid problems that accompany diabetes typically are elevated blood triglycerides, slightly elevated LDL cholesterol, and low HDL cholesterol.

Because type 2 diabetes is a clear and strong independent risk factor for developing CHD, people with diabetes need to pay particular attention to having their blood lipids checked frequently. If lipid abnormalities are present and you have diabetes, you'll need aggressive treatment to correct these problems.

Similarly, a common association exists between type 2 diabetes and obesity. Although not all diabetics are obese, more than 80 percent of all type 2 diabetics are overweight. If you have type 2 diabetes and you're overweight, the first and most important line of defense is losing weight.

Noting other conditions associated with cholesterol

Other medical conditions that may cause blood-lipid abnormalities include certain diseases of the kidney and liver and low thyroid levels. If you have any of these conditions, important steps to take include frequently checking your blood cholesterol and other lipid levels and discussing these issues in detail with your physician.

Considering severe and/or hereditary forms of elevated blood cholesterol

Approximately 1 to 2 percent of the populace of the U.S. has an inherited tendency for severely elevated blood cholesterol. These conditions typically result from genetic traits that affect how the body handles cholesterol. The best advice: If any member of your family has a severely elevated cholesterol level, you and all your family members need to consult with your physicians, be screened, and receive the proper therapy, if you have one of these genetic conditions.

Chapter 10

Managing Your Weight to Lower Your Risk

*I*f you are overweight or obese, one of the best things you can do to reduce multiple risk factors for heart disease is to lose weight. Losing as few as 5 to 10 percent of your body weight can make a significant difference. For many people that's just 10 to 15 pounds.

The major problem with being overweight is that those extra pounds not only represent an independent risk for developing heart disease but also increase other factors. For example, being overweight increases the risk of high blood pressure, the risk of higher LDL-cholesterol and triglycerides, and the risk of type 2 diabetes. The risk is also greater when the extra fat is in your abdominal area (apple shaped) rather than in your thighs and legs (pear-shaped) because that fat tends to be more metabolically active.

The good news is that losing just 5 to 10 percent of your overall weight (no matter where it is on your body) and maintaining that loss can reduce all these risk factors. Losing more weight if necessary to reach normal weight range can improve your health outlook even more. There's more good news: Adopting a heart-healthy diet and getting regular physical activity (Chapter 5) provide the foundation of reaching a healthier weight and maintaining it long-term. An effective weight-loss plan builds on these practices. This chapter provides proven techniques to help you succeed in reaching your goals.

Setting Realistic Weight-Loss Goals

Many forces in American culture drive us to desire instant satisfaction or accomplishment. But taking an "everything right now or nothing" approach to weight-loss (as to so many other things) is a recipe for failure and disappointment. For example, say that you hit the scales at 200 pounds at your last check up, and your doctor said, "For your height and age, you ought to weigh about 150 to 160 pounds." Groan. That's 40 to 50 pounds to lose — a real mountain to climb over in order to get down. The vision of months of deprivation is enough to stop you from even trying. Or maybe the news provokes you into trying an extreme diet that promises to take off 5 or 10 pounds a week. Either way, I can guarantee failure in your future.

A realistic weight-loss plan should be about discovery, not deprivation. That means that it should help you create new habits that are both enjoyable and healthful. So here are some tips for setting goals that work.

Recognize that your goal is adopting better habits for life

Losing weight is your measurable objective. But your primary goal is a healthier life, specifically a heart-healthy life. That means that the steps you must take to reach a healthier weight will be those that help you adopt healthier eating practices and a more active lifestyle for the long-term. Isn't this idea great? A weight-loss "diet" gives you a chance to enjoy delicious new foods and practice tasty, healthful cooking techniques.

Identify a reasonable weight-loss goal for 8 to 12 weeks

Extensive research suggests that most people can lose 1 to 2 pounds per week without sacrificing good nutrition or losing lean muscle mass. For most people, therefore, setting a goal of losing 5 percent of your weight in 12 weeks is a good initial goal. For example, say that your long-term target weight is 150 to 160 pounds. If you weigh 200 pounds, losing 5 percent would be 10 pounds. That means losing about a pound a week — a very doable target. A goal of 15 pounds would also be very doable — about 1.5 pounds per week. If you weigh 250 pounds, then 5 percent would be 12.5 pounds, also a very doable goal. If you weigh 175, then 5 percent would be about 8 to 9 pounds.

In all these cases, losing 5 percent of weight will bring health benefits and will achieve between a third and a half of your long-range goal within three months. The main plus is that research shows that most people can successfully lose up to 10 percent of their weight in six months; more important, people following this moderate pace are more likely to keep the weight off long-term.

Subdivide bigger challenges

If you need to lose larger amounts of weight, such as anything upwards of 20 pounds, then working on intermediate goals as described in the preceding section leads to greater success. After you've reached the goal for losing 5 percent of your weight, for example, then reset the goal to lose another 5 percent. Still keep your focus on choosing heart-healthy foods and developing healthful eating habits and staying physically active.

Take one step at a time

In many years of working with patients who are trying to lose weight, I have seen more people stumble because they tried to make too many changes at once than because they went more slowly and made one change at a time. If you "go for broke" by making lots of diet and lifestyle changes at the same time, you will almost certainly "crash and burn." You know what I mean: You dump the contents of the pantry and fridge and load up on new vegetables and whole grains you've never eaten, at least not often. You pile the fruit bowl with familiar and exotic fruits. You aim to cook one new recipe a meal. You schedule a 30 minute walk every day right away. The result? At the end of the first week, you are miserable, not to mention exhausted.

So when you develop your personal plan using the tips in the following sections, make changes one step at a time. You may even wish to first make some changes in the way you eat and start getting more physical activity before you begin to focus on weight loss.

Track your food intake and daily activities

Changing the way you eat and adding more physical activity to your day takes a big effort. After the excitement of making a positive start dims, boredom and even frustration can get in your way. A good way to keep yourself motivated is to keep track of your daily efforts. Numerous studies have shown this approach works.

There are various free online trackers and mobile apps. For example, Choosemyplate.gov, the website of the Dietary Guidelines for Americans, offers a reliable SuperTracker program that you can customize to your own plan and use online. Or you can set up your own spreadsheet or paper form.

Celebrate wins and forgive failures

When you achieve a small victory, such as losing 5 pounds, reward yourself. Just don't select food as the reward. Choose something else that you would like to do. Download a new book to your e-reader, take in a new movie, try a fun, new outdoor activity, and so on. Share this celebration with your family or friends.

There will always, however, be times in any new endeavor — including losing weight — when this old saying will seem to apply to your efforts: "The forwarder I go, the behinder I get." When that happens, don't worry about it. Forgive yourself. Start fresh the next day or, if you really lapsed, the next week. Your goal is to develop new habits that become second nature. That takes practice. Remind yourself that a lapse (or relapse) doesn't need to become a complete "collapse." Repeat that reminder frequently.

Involve family and/or friends

Support from family and friends for your weight-loss goals shores up your efforts. Because your weight-loss plan is based on heart-healthy eating, no special menus or foods are needed, and the whole family can participate. In many families, in fact, more than one person needs to lose weight. And everyone needs to eat in a heart-healthy way. Supporting each other can help everyone succeed in getting better nutrition and, if necessary, losing weight. If you are single, perhaps you have a friend or coworker who would like to partner with you, which can help keep both of you on track.

Developing Your Personal Weight-Loss Plan

In this section, I provide strategies for developing your own personal weight-loss plan. You can then use the strategies that work for you and your family to shape your specific plan. At a minimum, I suggest that you do the following:

✔ Write down overall goals for losing 5 to 10 percent of your body weight, or 10 to 20 pounds, over a 12 week or 3 month period. Select whichever weight goal is *lower*.

✔ Create specific objectives based on the strategies I outline in this section to help you reach these goals. For example, "add one vegetable to lunch and dinner each day" and "substitute whole grain hot or ready-to-eat cereal for toaster pastry for breakfast" are examples of two specific nutrition objectives. One week's physical activity objective if you are currently sedentary might be "walk 5 minutes briskly at least twice each day." The next week, you might increase your physical activity objective to "walk 10 minutes briskly at least once each day."

What this chapter does not give you is a specific diet that defines servings per day and gives you a meal plan. If you find daily meal plans helpful, I recommend several resources. But the goal is to empower yourself to make lasting changes in how you eat and live your life to support better well-being and prevent chronic disease, including heart disease and its risk factors.

Cutting calories — how low to go?

Hundreds of diets on the Internet and in the marketplace pitch "magic" strategies for quick loss. However, there's nothing magic about the basic fact of weight loss: To lose weight, you must burn more energy than you eat. There are two ways to do that — reduce the food calories you eat or burn up more calories than you eat with physical activity.

Extensive research has shown that if you use either of these strategies separately, you will typically lose more weight with diet alone than with exercise alone. However, the most successful losers in all types of studies with all types of diets have been individuals who combined a reduced calorie eating plan with regular physical activity or exercise. In fact, adding physical activity or exercise to a reduced calorie diet increases weight loss by about 20 percent over a diet alone.

Research has also shown that reducing your normal daily calorie intake by about 500 calories per day will result in losing between 1 and 2 pounds a week. No one should go lower than 1,200 calories daily, however, because it's hard to get the all the nutrients you need with very low-calorie intake.

Now, wait a minute — I can hear you saying — you said I wouldn't have to count calories. No, you don't have to do that. But it's helpful to know the parameters. Also, you may be among those who work best when you have some numbers to guide your planning. There are two basic numbers you may find most useful. First, what is your "normal" weight range? Second, what is the average daily calorie intake you need for someone of your gender, age, and activity level?

Figuring out where you stand, body-weight–wise

The quickest and most accurate way to get an idea of where you stand on the range of body weight is to use a Body Mass Index (BMI) table. Unless you do a lot of strength training and have a high lean muscle mass (like many athletes), then BMI will give you a good idea of where you are now and what goals you may wish to set. You can find a BMI calculator on the SuperTracker at ChooseMyPlate.gov.

Determining the number of calories you need

In terms of the appropriate daily calorie intake for you, the U.S. Department of Agriculture provides a detailed table (see Table 10-1).

This table, published by the U.S. Department of Health and Human Services and the U.S. Department of Agriculture, shows the estimated amounts of calories needed to maintain calorie balance for various gender and age groups at three different levels of physical activity. As you reference this table, keep these points in mind:

✔ The estimates are rounded to the nearest 200 calories. Your calorie needs may be higher or lower.

✔ The calorie estimates do not apply to pregnant or breastfeeding women.

✔ The activity levels indicate the following:

  • **Sedentary:** Only light physical activity associated with typical day-to-day life.

  • **Moderately Active:** Physical activity equivalent to walking 1.5 to 3 miles per day at 3 to 4 miles per hour in addition to the activities of daily living.

  • **Active:** Physical activity equivalent to walking more than 3 miles per day at 3 to 4 miles per hour in addition to the activities of daily living.

Table 10-1	Estimated Calorie Needs* per Day by Age, Gender, and Physical Activity					
	Male/ Sedentary	Male/ Moderately active	Male/ Active	Female/ Sedentary	Female/ Moderately active	Female/ Active
Age (years)						
2	1000	1000	1000	1000	1000	1000
3	1200	1400	1400	1000	1200	1400
4	1200	1400	1600	1200	1400	1400

	Male/ Sedentary	Male/ Moderately active	Male/ Active	Female/ Sedentary	Female/ Moderately active	Female/ Active
5	1200	1400	1600	1200	1400	1600
6	1400	1600	1800	1200	1400	1600
7	1400	1600	1800	1200	1600	1800
8	1400	1600	2000	1400	1600	1800
9	1600	1800	2000	1400	1600	1800
10	1600	1800	2200	1400	1800	2000
11	1800	2000	2200	1600	1800	2000
12	1800	2200	2400	1600	2000	2200
13	2000	2200	2600	1600	2000	2200
14	2000	2400	2800	1800	2000	2400
15	2200	2600	3000	1800	2000	2400
16	2400	2800	3200	1800	2000	2400
17	2400	2800	3200	1800	2000	2400
18	2400	2800	3200	1800	2000	2400
19-20	2600	2800	3000	2000	2200	2400
21-25	2400	2800	3000	2000	2200	2400
26-30	2400	2600	3000	1800	2000	2400
31-35	2400	2600	3000	1800	2000	2200
36-40	2400	2600	2800	1800	2000	2200
41-45	2200	2600	2800	1800	2000	2200
46-50	2200	2400	2800	1800	2000	2200
51-55	2200	2400	2800	1600	1800	2200
56-60	2200	2400	2600	1600	1800	2200
61-65	2000	2400	2600	1600	1800	2000
67-70	2000	2200	2600	1600	1800	2000
71-75	2000	2200	2600	1600	1800	2000
76+	2000	2200	2400	1600	1800	2000

* Calorie levels are based on the Estimated Energy Requirements (EER) and activity levels from the Institute of Medicine Dietary Reference Intakes for Energy and Macronutrients, 2002.
Source: Appendix 6. Dietary Guidelines for Americans, 2010.

Considering a specific eating plan

If you prefer a structured eating plan rather than creating your own using the strategies I share in the next section, then I recommend either the DASH eating plan or the Mediterranean diet. Although created to help lower blood pressure, the DASH eating plan has a track record as one of the best weight-loss eating plans, also. You can download a PDF of the booklet *Lowering Your Blood Pressure with DASH* (`http://www.nhlbi.nih.gov/health/resources/heart/hbp-dash-index.htm`) that gives you the information you need. The booklet describes the eating plan, provides servings per day at different calorie levels and gives a week of daily meal plans.

The general eating pattern known as the Mediterranean diet has also served as the basis for many diet plans. I recommend the weight-loss approach found in the *Mediterranean Diet Cookbook for Dummies*, by Meri Raffetto and Wendy Jo Peterson, who are registered dietitians. Some of their great recipes are also featured in Part IV of this book.

Selecting how many meals and snacks daily

If you are trying to lose weight, should you stick to eating just three meals a day, or is snacking allowed? The answer actually varies because you need to choose what works best for you and keeps you feeling satisfied and not deprived. I can tell you that among a national registry of people who lost a significant amount of weight and kept it off, most ate three meals and two snacks daily. Interestingly, that's also the most common eating pattern among the general population. Whatever your preferred eating pattern, you can make choices that increase your nutrient intake and lower your energy intake.

Controlling portions the easy way

Supersizing portions has crept into our homes as well as into packaged foods and restaurant meals. Interesting research, such as the many studies done by Dr. Brian Wansink or Dr. Barbara Rolls, have shown that there are a number of techniques that you can use to resize your portions to sensible quantities without having to remember a lot of measurement equivalents. Here are just a few tips gleaned from their studies and others:

✔ **Use smaller plates for meals.** If your plate is 10 inches in diameter rather than 12 inches — or even 8 or 9 inches rather than 10 inches — you will typically place smaller portions on them.

✔ **Use a tall, skinny glass rather than a short wide glass.** Studies have shown that people pour more and drink more when they use a short, wide glass.

✔ **Serve plates in the kitchen, not at the table.** Serving plates in the kitchen rather than placing serving bowls on the table allows portion control. Refrigerate leftovers before dining to avoid the temptation of second servings.

✔ **Serve a salad before the meal.** Dress it with low-calorie, low-fat dressing, of course. Studies show that eating a salad before the main meal reduces overall calorie intake. Two or three cups of salad greens also help you feel full and satisfied. A clear broth soup (not cream) with vegetables and no meat can also play this role.

The best salads to use feature nutritious greens and raw vegetables, such as carrots, tomatoes, peppers, squash, cucumber, jicama, and the like. You get lots of nutrients for very few calories.

✔ **Keep single-serving packets of snacks on hand.** When the munchies hit, having a portion-controlled single serving packet of a nutritious food in the pantry can keep you from overeating right out of the box. Single serving low-fat microwave popcorn is a good example of a prepackaged whole grain snack; 5 cups of popped popcorn have about 100 calories. If you can't do without sweet or savory treats, portion-controlled packets can help you keep a handle on this indulgence.

Make your own 100 to 120 calorie packets of whole grain ready-to-eat cereal, trail mix, or nuts. Reusable containers or baggies work fine.

Substituting nutrient-rich foods and techniques for the energy-dense

At every meal or snack you have an opportunity to select foods that have a higher nutrient value over ones that have more energy (calories) and fewer nutrients. Making such substitutions is the basic technique for achieving a heart-healthy way of eating and for losing those pounds. Here are some basic approaches.

✔ **Make vegetables and fruits the main features of lunch and dinner.** Fruits and vegetables are generally high in nutrients and low in calories, particularly if you season them with herbs, lemon juice, or butter sprinkles rather than butter or margarine. Using a little flavorful, healthy oil, such as olive oil or walnut oil, is not low-calorie but does add nutrients. Choose smaller portions of starchy vegetables such as potatoes or corn and smaller portions of lean meat, such as chicken, or seafood.

✔ **Use cooking methods that don't add calories.** Steaming, boiling, baking, and roasting add no calories. Sautéing and stir frying use just a little oil; in fact, using a cooking spray adds almost none. If you need moisture, water, vegetable stock, or low-fat chicken stock will often work well. Avoid pan frying and deep frying. For example, select a baked potato with nonfat yogurt or new potatoes dressed with a dash of olive oil, lemon juice, and parsley over french fries. Try oven-baked crispy chicken rather than fried chicken.

✔ **Add vegetables to main dishes.** Lower the calories in popular dishes like spaghetti, chili, lasagna, and even pizza by adding vegetables. For example, add diced carrots, celery, and peppers along with kernel corn and beans to chili. Tomatoes and spinach work well in macaroni and cheese. Make your Irish stew a quarter lean beef cubes and three quarters carrots, onions, tomatoes, and potatoes.

✔ **Enjoy a meatless meal two or three days per week.** Go Mediterranean at dinner with Ratatouille (see Chapter 18 for the recipe), whole grain bread, and fruit. Or enjoy a primavera spaghetti — fresh or canned diced tomatoes, carrots, peppers, asparagus, onions, garlic, and yellow or zucchini squash, sautéed with a little olive oil (1 teaspoon oil to 1 cup vegetables) for the sauce, served over wholegrain pasta and topped with 1 tablespoon per serving of grated Parmesan or pecorino cheese. For lunch, enjoy raw vegetables and whole grain pita bread with classic hummus (you can find a recipe in Chapter 19), or select the Black Beans with Tomatoes and Feta recipe in Chapter 17 and add some fruit.

✔ **Focus breakfast on whole grains, fruit, and low-fat dairy.** Select oatmeal (rolled or steel cut, not instant) for a hot cereal. (Make enough for several days by cooking it overnight in a slow cooker). For speed, enjoy whole-grain ready-to-eat cereal (low in added sugar) with fruit (blueberries, strawberries, raisins) and topped with low-fat or non-diary milk. Instead of a big bagel, select a whole grain English muffin or Mark's Low-Fat Oat Bran Muffins with Peaches (Chapter 16) to eat with low-fat yogurt and fruit. Enjoy an occasional egg but skip the sausage and bacon. For a weekend brunch, try one of our heart-healthy breakfast recipes, such as Eggs Benedict with Asparagus and Low-Fat Hollandaise, which you can find in Chapter 16.

Snacking for better nutrition

The right snack when you get a little hungry can keep you from eating more than you intend later. So I advise keeping nutritious snacks readily available. Here are some of my family's favorites:

✓ **Fresh fruit.** Keep a bowl of apples, oranges, tangerines, and pears ready to eat on the kitchen counter. Keep perishable fruit such as grapes or strawberries washed, portioned, and ready in the refrigerator. Melons, such as cantaloupe, honeydew, and watermelon, can be chunked and refrigerated in a closed container; melon will stay fresh to eat for two to four days if you don't combine it with other fruit.

✓ **Greek yogurt.** Non-fat Greek yogurt is full of protein and easy to mix with berries or other fruit.

✓ **Peanut butter.** Low-sodium, natural peanut butter goes well with whole-grain bread, apple slices, or bananas. It's a good source of protein and healthful oils.

✓ **Popcorn.** Air-popped or low-fat microwave popcorn is whole grain and satisfies the desire for a crunchy snack. Just don't douse it in melted butter.

✓ **Nuts.** A handful of nuts (1 to 2 ounces) is nutritious and delicious. Choose dry roasted peanuts over oil roasted. Eat almonds, pecans, or walnuts raw or roasted. I divide bigger containers into single serving baggies to prevent overindulging — it's hard to stop with just one handful of nuts because they taste so good!

✓ **Dry cereal or homemade trail mix.** Kids love a mix of whole-grain ready-to-eat cereals as a snack. Pack a cup of a single cereal or a mix into reusable containers. (Select those that are low in sodium and added sugar.) Add a few raisins and nuts to make your own trail mix.

One of the best ways to avoid eating too much of a snack is never to eat straight out of the bag or box. That tip applies no matter how "righteous" the snack — baby carrots, anyone?

Brown-bagging your lunch

Lunch is the meal that Americans most often eat in restaurants (though breakfast is catching up). One of the ways that you can make lunch work positively toward your weight-loss goals is to bring your own healthful lunch from home rather than eat out. For days that you are too busy to make a lunch, keep a few single-serving frozen meals on hand; many companies today are making calorie- and portion-controlled meals that feature vegetables and lean protein. Check the labels for sodium and fat content before you choose.

If you dine out, you can still make lunch weight-loss friendly. First, choose a restaurant that works for you. Then, make healthier choices. For example, rather than a broiled chicken sandwich, choose a salad with broiled chicken on top. Ask for dressing on the side and dip your fork in the dressing before picking up a bite. Get a half sandwich rather than a large whole sandwich, and choose lean ingredients and whole-grain bread; dress the sandwich with mustard rather than mayonnaise. No half sandwiches? Then take off one slice of bread and make it "open face."

Adding Regular Physical Activity

As I noted earlier, you will usually have more success with your weight-loss plan if you add regular physical activity. The activity that's most accessible to most people is walking. All you need to begin with a single step out your front door are good shoes and comfortable clothing. I discuss how to get started in Chapter 5.

If you have health issues or are significantly overweight, it's a good idea to check with your doctor before beginning an exercise program. But remember, if you have been sedentary, you are going to start with small sessions of walking and gradually increase both the length of time you walk and the intensity at which you walk. For some health issues, your doctor may want you to keep your heart rate within a certain target range; Chapter 5 discusses how to do that using an inexpensive heart rate monitor.

At this point you may be wondering, how many calories does physical activity burn? That depends on the intensity of the exercise. In general, the more vigorous the intensity, the more calories burned in a given time. For example, aerobic dance or Zumba performed at vigorous intensity for 30 minutes burns more calories than 30 minutes of moderate-intensity walking. However, if you have not been active, you shouldn't try to plunge right into vigorous activity. Work up to it. Remember, every bit of moderate activity helps you burn more calories than sitting at your computer on in your easy chair before the TV.

One easy way to increase moderate activity throughout your day is to wear a pedometer (you can get good ones for less than $10), and increase the steps you take each day. Try to add 100 to 200 steps every couple of days. Set an end goal of 10,000 steps a day. Without realizing it, you'll find that you are climbing stairs rather than taking the elevator, taking any parking place no matter how far from the store, mowing the lawn cheerfully, and even walking to do nearby errands. If you hit 10,000 steps daily, you may not need another aerobic exercise activity.

What about boredom?

Most people can mix and match activities without spending a fortune on gym or health club memberships. Here are some suggestions if your activity is walking:

✔ Plan out different walking routes and ask a family member or friend to walk with you; conversation makes the time pass pleasantly. Committing to walk with someone also keeps you accountable.

✔ Include several activities. For example, walk on some days and bicycle on others. If you have a swimming pool available, add swimming on a couple of days. Take a yoga or tai chi class on some days — many community centers offer such classes for moderate fees.

✔ Train for a walking, running, or cycling event that supports a charity you care about. That's great motivation.

Don't neglect strength training

Lean muscle mass not only burns calories, but it also helps people stay functionally fit and able to safely perform all the activities of daily living. For those reasons, it's important to maintain and even build lean muscle mass when you are trying to lose weight. Aerobic activity strengthens muscles to a degree, but actively building muscle requires resistance training.

Most people think of resistance training as weight lifting. However, many other types of exercise also provide resistance and build muscle. Swimming and water aerobics, for example, are two exercises that provide both aerobic and strength training. Yoga provides strength training by using the body's own weight as resistance. Calisthenic exercises also use the body's weight and opposing muscle groups to provide resistance that builds muscle. All these are options you may wish to explore.

Taking Time for Yourself

You won't find this objective in many weight-loss programs, but I think it's important. Why are you working to lose weight? Because you want a healthier, better life, right? An important part of a better life, in my experience, is taking time for activities that refresh your spirit. Maybe that's spending more time with your spouse doing something just the two of you want to do. Maybe it's taking time off with your family. Perhaps volunteering for a cause you support gives you a boost. For many patients I've worked with, taking time to garden each day makes them feel connected to life and the future. Taking time to invest in activities meaningful to you will provide "something more" that helps you keep going forward with your weight-loss goals.

Chapter 11

Quitting Smoking

. . . .

. . . .

*O*nly one good thing can be said about cigarette smoking — it's good when you stop! In the United States, cigarette smoking is responsible for an enormous amount of unnecessary suffering and death every year:

✔ Cigarette smoking is the leading cause of preventable death in the U.S., claiming more than 430,000 lives per year.

✔ Depending on the amount of cigarette smoking you do, it increases your risk of heart disease between 200 percent and 400 percent.

✔ Smoking increases your risk of lung cancer by 15 to 30 times.

✔ Smoking harms the people around you through secondhand smoke, which increases the risk of heart disease and lung cancer in nonsmokers and may result in chronic bronchitis in children who live with smokers.

But guess what? None of this information is news to people who smoke cigarettes. As a friend of mine once said, "Everyone who doesn't exercise knows that they should, and everyone who smokes cigarettes knows that they shouldn't!"

So I'm not going to rattle off too many statistics about why you need to stop smoking. Instead, I simply review enough about how smoking relates to coronary heart disease to give your willpower extra ammunition against the urges of your nicotine habit or to reinforce your commitment to supporting someone who's trying to quit. After that, I discuss some specific recommendations for *how to* stop smoking. For the good of your heart and overall health, it's never too late to quit.

Affirming Reasons for Not Smoking

Cigarette smoke harms virtually every vital organ, but it is particularly dangerous to the heart and lungs. Incidentally, anyone who thinks they're safe using smokeless tobacco, cigars, or pipes needs to think again. More about going smokeless in the section "Reviewing the Dangers of Other Forms of Tobacco" later in the chapter.

Linking cigarette smoking and heart disease

As a cardiologist, I'm astounded that so many people still don't appreciate just how serious the link is between cigarette smoking and heart disease.

Depending on how much they smoke, cigarette smokers increase their risk of developing heart disease two to four times more than nonsmokers. In fact, every cigarette that you light up increases your blood pressure, and the nicotine you take in causes coronary arteries to mildly constrict (close down). This problem is bad enough in a normal person, but for someone who suffers with angina, it can bring on significant symptoms. Smoking also increases inflammation and damage to artery walls, making it easier for artery-narrowing plaque to form.

In addition, cigarette smoking decreases the good cholesterol (HDL) in your bloodstream and increases the bad cholesterol (LDL). It also significantly increases your risk of developing peripheral vascular disease and aortic disease (which affects the main blood vessel leaving the heart).

Linking cigarette smoking with other diseases

Smoking accounts for many cancer deaths in the U.S., including 90 percent of lung cancer deaths. Smoking also is associated with cancers of the mouth and throat, esophagus, pancreas, cervix, kidney, and bladder. Want more bad news? Cigarette smoking is associated with such annoying, chronic conditions as the common cold, stomach ulcers, chronic bronchitis, and many other lung diseases, and with catastrophic events, such as stroke.

Considering smoking and women

For reasons that aren't completely clear, cigarette smoking appears to be particularly dangerous for women. Smoking causes 60 percent of heart attacks in women younger than age 50. Combining smoking and oral contraceptives increases the risk of a heart attack by 40 percent. One possible explanation for this increased risk for women is the interaction between the chemicals in cigarette smoke and female hormones. In addition, lung cancer is now the leading cause of cancer death in women in the U.S., having surpassed breast cancer in 1987.

Considering smoking and children

More than 90 percent of current smokers started when they were children. Sadly, every day an estimated 3,200 children younger than 18 smoke their first cigarettes, and 2,000 of these youngsters will become regular smokers. Although teen cigarette smoking has declined substantially since 2000, over 23 percent of high school students currently use tobacco products: 14 percent smoke cigarettes, 12.6 percent smoke cigars, and 6.4 percent use smokeless tobacco. One third to one half of teens use more than one tobacco product.

If you never start smoking as a child, however, you're unlikely ever to start smoking. If you're a young smoker, the best thing you can do for your long-term good health is kick the tobacco habit now.

Considering smoking and African Americans

Cigarette smoking also appears particularly dangerous for African Americans. One reasons may be that African Americans are 1.5 times more likely to have multiple risk factors for coronary heart disease (CHD). Most prominent are high blood pressure, diabetes, and obesity. In addition 75 percent of African American smokers prefer menthol cigarettes, which enable quicker absorption of nicotine and its byproducts into the blood. For these reasons and others that aren't completely clear, African Americans who smoke appear more susceptible to heart disease than other groups of Americans.

Considering the dangers of secondhand smoke

People who live or work with active cigarette smokers are susceptible to *secondhand smoke* (also called *passive smoke, environmental tobacco smoke,* or *ETS*), which enters the air from lighted cigarettes or the exhalations of smokers. Every year, about 34,000 deaths from heart disease and over 7,000 deaths from lung cancer are attributed to secondhand smoke. Secondhand smoke also is responsible for between 150,000 and 300,000 respiratory tract infections annually.

Checking out the benefits of quitting

Before you get too depressed about all the bad news associated with cigarette smoking, take a look at the bright side:

✔ In the U.S., about 50 million citizens are successful former smokers. After only one year of not smoking, the excess cardiac risk from smoking is cut in half. Fifteen years after you stop smoking, your risk is similar to that of a person who never smoked.

✔ Smokers who quit between age 35 and 44 gain an average of 9 years in life expectancy. Quitting between 45 and 54 gains a former smoker about 6 years in longevity. Even men and women who quit between the ages of 65 and 69 can increase their life expectancies, not to mention improve their health. In one recent study, 65-year-old women who quit smoking added an average of four years to their life expectancies.

✔ Quitting smoking is truly possible. With modern smoking cessation programs, 20 percent to 40 percent of participants successfully stop smoking. Aids now in the marketplace that help people quit smoking may help this success rate climb even higher.

Understanding Nicotine Addiction: A Chain That Binds

Nicotine is a powerfully addictive drug. Using nicotine causes changes in the brain that compel people to use it more and more. In addition, attempting to stop using nicotine causes unpleasant physical and emotional side effects. Good feelings when the drug is present combined with bad feelings when the drug is not present are the hallmarks of addiction. And many researchers judge nicotine to be as addicting as heroin and cocaine.

Examining what nicotine does to the body

When you smoke a cigarette, ingesting the chemical nicotine causes a number of immediate responses in your body. In the short term, your blood pressure and heart rate rise, and the arteries supplying your heart narrow. When these arteries narrow, the combination of nicotine and carbon monoxide absorbed from the smoke spell double trouble to your heart, because carbon monoxide reduces the amount of oxygen that the blood can carry. In addition, smoking causes abnormalities in the way that your body handles various fats, causing a decrease in the good cholesterol (HDL) and an increase in the bad cholesterol (LDL). It also affects various hormones and how the body handles blood sugar.

Understanding nicotine's impact on the heart

Cigarette smoking harms the heart and the arteries. Carbon monoxide in cigarette smoke appears to damage the walls of arteries and encourages the buildup of fat along these walls. Nicotine may also contribute to this process. In addition, chemicals in cigarette smoke make blood platelets stickier and thereby increase the likelihood that your blood will clot. All these effects combined significantly increase the risk of heart disease.

Checking out nicotine replacement products

Many smokers who want to quit turn to *nicotine replacement products* such as nicotine transdermal patches, nicotine gum and lozenges, and nicotine nasal spray and inhalers. These products have been successful in helping smokers quit when they're used as part of an comprehensive program to quit smoking. Nicotine, of course, is still nicotine, and it's still addictive. But nicotine replacement is different from smoking in at least two important physical ways:

- ✔ First, when using nicotine replacements, you avoid inhaling harmful carbon monoxide, tars, and other toxins that are present in smoke.

- ✔ Second, when you smoke, nicotine is delivered to your brain in a sudden rush that tapers off over a couple of hours. Nicotine replacements deliver nicotine to your body at a steadier rate or lower rate.

Getting away from that hit of nicotine may make quitting easier. At any rate, such nicotine substitutions appear to help ease some of the psychological and physiological problems associated with withdrawal from nicotine. In an optimal situation, you should work with your doctor when using nicotine replacement therapy, even though nicotine patches and gum now are available over the counter.

If you're diagnosed with any form of heart disease, never use any nicotine replacement product or e-cigarette (which I discuss in the next section) without discussing it with your physician. In general, unsupervised nicotine-replacement therapy is not recommended for patients with heart or circulatory problems.

Weighing in on e-cigs

What about e-cigarettes? Many users say that quitting smoking is why they tried the e-cigarette, and most brands advertise that purpose. However, the scientific jury is still out on whether e-cigarettes are actually helpful to many individuals in quitting smoking. In addition, the limited research to date on the safety of e-cigarettes is inconclusive. The many different types of e-cigarette vary substantially in what amounts of nicotine they may deliver and what additives and potential toxins they contain in addition to nicotine.

Using a plain e-cigarette (no exotic flavors or additives) for the short term is undoubtedly safer than smoking tobacco. But there has not been time for long-term studies yet, and unlike nicotine replacement products, e-cigarettes are not yet regulated.

Reviewing the Dangers of Other Forms of Tobacco

Although this chapter focuses mainly on cigarette smoking, no form of tobacco is safe. Here's a look at some of the other forms of tobacco use:

- **Smokeless tobacco:** The use of all forms of smokeless tobacco, including plug, leaf, and snuff, has remained popular, particularly among men, according to recent data. Such products often are referred to as *spit tobacco.* Perhaps the greatest cause for concern is the highly addictive practice of *dipping snuff,* which is when tobacco (either moist leaf snuff or dry powdered snuff) is placed between the cheek and the gum. Nicotine and other cancer-causing agents are absorbed through the gum tissues and expose the body to levels of nicotine equal to those of cigarette smoking. The nicotine from smokeless tobacco poses dangers similar to those from cigarettes. In addition, individuals who dip snuff have a greatly increased risk of developing mouth and throat cancers, which are among the most difficult to treat effectively.

- ✔ **Cigars:** What price glitter and phony sophistication? Although the sale of expensive cigars isn't growing as fast as it was during the 1990s, sales of cigars have continued to grow. Regardless of the elitist, stylish image hyped in slick magazines, cigar smoking is extremely hazardous to your health. Almost all the same cancer-causing agents found in cigarettes also are found in cigars. But the overall death rate is increased by almost 40 percent in individuals who smoke cigars when compared with non-smokers. The increased risk of mouth cancers is between 500 percent and 1,000 percent. Oh, so you don't inhale the smoke? Well then, exactly what is that blue haze hanging about that trendy smoker's bar or your living room?

- ✔ **Pipe smoking:** Although less data is available about smoking pipes than cigars, there is no reason to doubt that pipes are just as dangerous as cigars. Pipe smokers certainly experience increased cancers of the lip and mouth.

Taking Steps to Stop Smoking

One of the first things you need to do when you decide to quit smoking is set up a firm foundation for a successful campaign by considering the following guidelines. These tips are based on reviews of plenty of research, and they're consistent with the recommendations for quitting from a number of health agencies:

- ✔ **Be committed.** Breaking the nicotine addiction isn't easy. It takes an enormous individual effort. But you can be encouraged by the fact that half the people who ever smoked cigarettes have quit.

- ✔ **Talk to your doctor.** Ask your physician about nicotine replacement therapy and other available programs to help you quit smoking. This type of communication helps maximize your chances of success.

- ✔ **Set a quit date.** Studies show that you're more likely to stop smoking if you set a specific date instead of trying to taper off.

- ✔ **Build on past mistakes.** The average cigarette smoker usually tries to quit smoking six to ten times before doing so successfully. Review what has worked and what has not worked for you during past efforts.

- ✔ **Seek the support of family and friends.** Tell your family and friends that you're trying to quit smoking and enlist them in your efforts to stop. If they're truly your friends, they'll be supportive.

- ✔ **Learn how to cope.** Most cigarette smoking is triggered by other cues. Try minimizing or working around the cues in your life that stimulate you to smoke.

✔ **Take the focus off weight gain.** True, many people who stop smoking gain some weight, but the vast majority of them gain fewer than ten pounds. The health benefits of quitting smoking far outweigh the risks of the small weight gain that some people experience when they stop.

✔ **Avoid dieting while trying to stop smoking.** Remember that famous slogan for success: KISS! (Keep it simple, stupid!) Trying to change too many things at once is an invitation for failure.

Using Helpful Aids to Stop Smoking

A number of different options are available to help you stop smoking. Recent research shows that three particular program elements are particularly effective when used either alone or together to help smokers quit:

✔ **Nicotine replacement therapy:** Using nicotine replacement products, such as nicotine patches, gum, lozenges, inhalers, and nasal spray, increases the likelihood of quitting successfully. Nicotine patches, gum, and lozenges can now be obtained without a prescription. Nicotine nasal sprays and inhalers also have been approved by the Food and Drug Administration (FDA) and may be helpful for some individuals. Also talk to your doctor about some of the non-nicotine prescription medications that are now available.

✔ **Social support:** Receiving encouragement and support from your physician and your family is important. Support from others who are trying to quit smoking may also be helpful. Various smoking cessation groups are sure to be meeting in your area (community-based and commercial). And you may even want to try an online support group like the one that QuitNet (http://www.quitnet.com) provides.

For other online groups and resources type in "smoking cessation" as the search term on your web browser. Although that term sounds a bit stiff and technical, you'll probably get the best results with it. I also provide additional resources at the end of this chapter.

✔ **Skills training/problem-solving:** Listening to the practical advice and techniques that physicians, other healthcare workers, smoking-cessation specialists, and people who've quit can provide is extremely helpful when you're trying to quit smoking. Many states now have telephone *quit lines* you can call to speak with a counselor about your plan and available resources. Group and individual counseling also can help. Counseling needs to be intensive and last for at least two weeks but preferably up to eight weeks.

Other techniques that may help you quit smoking include acupuncture and hypnosis. In all instances, these aids should be used in conjunction with a comprehensive program prescribed by your physician and/or smoking cessation specialist.

Developing a Specific Plan to Quit

A variety of sources offer excellent information to help smokers break the habit. Some particularly helpful resources were developed by the National Cancer Institute (NCI — your tax dollars at work in a good cause). You can review these resources online at `http://www.smokefree.gov`.

Here are key recommendations adapted from the National Cancer Institute materials:

- **Prepare yourself to quit.** After you decide to quit, list all the reasons why you want to quit, and get yourself ready. Set a target date for quitting, perhaps a special day such as a birthday, or anniversary, or the Great American Smokeout, which takes place annually on the third Thursday in November.

- **Know what to expect.** Be realistic. You're going to experience some withdrawal symptoms, but they usually last only one to two weeks.

- **Involve someone else.** Get the support of your family, friends, and physician. Maybe even ask another smoker to quit with you. You can't overestimate the importance of support.

- **Before your quit day, you may want to prepare yourself with these techniques:**

  - Switch brands. Find one that you find distasteful.

  - Cut down the number of cigarettes that you smoke each day.

  - Try not to smoke automatically (after meals and during phone calls, for example).

  - Make smoking inconvenient. Go outside to smoke when it's cold or raining, go to malls or movies where smoking is prohibited, and so on.

  - Clean your clothes to get rid of the smell of cigarettes.

- **On the day that you quit, use these strategies:**

  - Throw away all your cigarettes, matches, and lighters; if you can't stand to throw away your collection of ashtrays, store them in the most inaccessible corner of your attic.

- Keep busy with plenty of activities on the big quit day. Remind your family and friends so that they can be extra supportive.

- Think about things that you'd like to buy for yourself. Estimate their cost in terms of packs of cigarettes and put aside the money to buy these presents.

- At the end of the day, buy yourself a treat or celebrate.

✔ **Immediately after you quit, adopt these techniques:**

- Develop a clean, fresh nonsmoking environment. Buy flowers now that you can enjoy their scents.

- Drink large quantities of water.

- If you miss the sensation of having a cigarette in your hand, find something else to keep your hands and fingers occupied.

- Look for ways to minimize your temptation and to develop new habits, such as exercise. Exercising decreases yet another risk factor for heart disease.

- Don't worry about gaining a small amount of weight, but do make sure that you have a well-balanced diet. As the appetite-depressing effect of nicotine disappears, avoid replacing cigarettes with calorie-dense candy, cookies, and snack foods. Try sugar-free gum or fresh fruits instead. Doing so helps you deal with the common experience of gaining some weight after you stop smoking.

Relapsing is not collapsing

If you slip and start to smoke again, don't be discouraged or give up. Remember, most smokers have to try several times before they finally succeed at quitting. Don't be too hard on yourself, and get back on the nonsmoking track as quickly as possible.

Quitting for keeps

As you keep the faith — and fight the good fight — not smoking eventually becomes a part of you. You develop your own techniques and strategies for sustaining the positive feeling and pride that having stopped smoking gives you. Remaining vigilant about what triggers your smoking urge is important for a long time after you quit. When that old urge kicks in, make a mental note about what was going on when it happened. What were you doing? Where were you? Who were you with? What were you thinking? Check off the things that may trigger you to want to smoke and try counteracting them with specific strategies. Never give up — you can do it!

Finding More Information

Many different resources are available to help you in your fight to stop smoking. Here are a few organizations and websites:

- **Smokefree.gov,** a project of the Nation Cancer Institute, provides great information. You can find a comprehensive guide to quitting, look up local and state quit line phone numbers, and talk to experts via e-mail. Phone: 877-44U-QUIT. Check out special sites for teens (`www.teen.smokefree.gov`), women (`www.women.smokefree.gov`) and Spanish speakers (`http://www.espanol.smokefree.gov`)

- **BeTobaccoFree.gov,** a project of the Department of Health and Human services, offers information, mobile apps, and other aids to quitting. Website: `betobaccofree.hhs.gov`.

- **Nicotine Anonymous** conducts a 12-step support program. Use its website (`www.nicotine-anonymous.org`) to locate meetings or find literature.

- **The American Heart Association** offers resources about why and how to quit, statistics about smoking, and articles about smoking's effects on your body. Website: `http://www.heart.org`.

- **The American Lung Association** has a popular quit-smoking course that's now available as a seven-module, interactive, online course. Look for "Freedom from Smoking Online" under the "Stop Smoking" Button on the ALA homepage. Website: `http://www.lung.org`.

- **The American Cancer Association** also has resources to help you quit smoking. Just enter "quit smoking" in the Association's website's search function. Website: `http://www.cancer.org`.

Part IV
Treating Heart Disease

5 Lifestyle Steps to Lower Your Risk of Needing Heart Treatment

- **Lose weight or maintain a healthy weight.** Because being overweight is an independent risk factor for heart disease and usually contributes to high blood pressure, elevated cholesterol, and type 2 diabetes, losing weight if you are overweight and maintaining a healthy weight can help decrease your risk of heart disease. Losing weight may also reduce your need for certain medications for blood pressure or cholesterol.

- **Stay active.** Getting at least 150 minutes weekly of moderate-intensity physical activity promotes cardiovascular fitness. This amount of physical activity is also associated with lower blood pressure, better cholesterol levels, and greater insulin sensitivity — all of which lower your risk of heart disease and needing medications or other therapies.

- **Eat a Mediterranean or DASH diet.** Eating a diet that features lots of vegetables, fruits, whole grains, nuts, lean or plant-based protein, healthy oils such as olive oil, and low-fat dairy has been associated with lower rates of risk factors for heart disease such as high blood pressure, elevated cholesterol, and type 2 diabetes. The Mediterranean Diet and the Dash Diet (see Chapter 5) are great examples of this approach to heart-healthy eating.

- **Get plenty of sleep.** Sleep has been associated with better overall health, increased longevity, and lower risk of heart disease. For most adults, "plenty of sleep" means getting seven to nine hours.

- **Share a little love.** People who stay connected with family and friends have better health and greater longevity than those who are alone or isolated. Volunteers who give back to the community also have better health outcomes, even if they have heart disease.

Find reliable information online about heart medications, tests, and procedures by using this guide at www.dummies.com/extras/preventingreversing heartdisease.

In this part . . .

✔ Look at the most common drug and medical treatments (short of invasive or surgical procedures) that are available to physicians for treating various heart problems and risk factors.

✔ Investigate the most common invasive procedures, such as angioplasty, and surgical procedures, such as coronary bypass grafting, that are used to treat heart problems.

✔ Investigate complementary therapies that may be helpful in preventing and controlling heart disease and discover others that could put you at risk.

✔ Find out why cardiac rehab is one of the best ways you can take back your life and health after a diagnosis of heart disease, a heart attack, or some other heart event and what to expect from cardiac rehabilitation programs.

Chapter 12

Modern Medical Arsenal: Rx Weapons for Heart Disease

*A*t first glance, the term *medical arsenal* probably suggests drugs or medications to most people. Would it surprise you to know that medical treatment is any therapy that is not surgical? Although this chapter's discussion focuses primarily on medications used in the treatment of the more common risk factors and manifestations of heart disease, it is important to remember that healthful lifestyle modifications and practices are the foundation of medical therapy for heart disease and its risk factors. Drugs and other medical treatments are used in conjunction with lifestyle measures, not in place of them.

In this chapter, I first discuss medical therapies for several risk factors for heart disease and then for some manifestations of heart disease, such as angina, heart attack, and heart failure.

Because many heart conditions are interrelated and affect each other, you will notice that many heart medications may be used to treat more than one condition. If you have one or more risk factors or heart conditions and need medication, remember to keep working with your doctor to be sure that your medicines are adjusted to best meet your needs and well-being.

Medically Treating Cardiac Risk Factors

Among major risk factors for heart disease, high blood pressure and cholesterol problems (dyslipidemias) are two major risk factors that are directly linked to the development of coronary heart disease (CHD). When lifestyle measures fail to control blood pressure and lipid problems, your doctor will choose from a variety of effective medications to create a treatment regimen that is appropriate for you. Diabetes and stress are two more major risk factors that may also be treated with medications as well as other techniques when necessary.

As discussed in Chapter 3, three additional important risk factors — physical inactivity, obesity, and a poor diet — have a direct effect on the risk factors named in the preceding paragraph, as well as on heart health and overall health. In general, you can address inactivity, obesity, and poor diet primarily with lifestyle modifications.

It's important to remember that the risk factors for CHD don't exist in isolation but interact to affect heart health and your overall wellness.

Lowering high blood pressure

Medicines are definitely indicated whenever positive lifestyle measures haven't succeeded in adequately lowering your blood pressure (see Chapter 8 for more details on high blood pressure). In this situation, your physician has many excellent medications to choose from.

Different medications, however, work differently for different individuals. So a period of adjustment may be needed to find out just which medication or combination of medications works best for you. The latest treatment guidelines note that most individuals require two or more medications used simultaneously to reach blood pressure goals. If your doctor needs to combine several medications, they often will come from different classes.

The following general classes of medications typically are used in controlling high blood pressure.

- ✔ **Diuretics:** Diuretics are the oldest blood pressure medication and the least expensive. Many guidelines recommend them as the first choice for hypertension. Diuretics work by lowering blood volume through increasing the amount of sodium and water passed through the kidneys. They also have a direct beneficial effect on the blood vessels, helping to lower blood pressure. Because diuretics typically increase urination, they are popularly known as *water pills.* If you have other medical conditions, such as diabetes, your doctor may prescribe a different first medication. Diuretics are often combined with another drug such as a beta blocker or ACE inhibitor (see the following categories).

- ✔ **Beta blockers and alpha blockers:** These medications work by blocking the effect of the hormones norepinephrine (noradrenaline) and epinephrine (adrenaline). As a result, the heart beats more slowly and with less force and the arteries relax or dilate — actions that lower blood pressure. Beta blockers are another popular first choice as treatment for high blood pressure for many patients. Depending on a your particular conditions and experience of side effects, however, your doctor might choose an alpha blocker first, or a combination beta and alpha blocker.

✔ **ACE inhibitors:** These drugs help reduce blood pressure by decreasing substances in the blood that cause vessels to constrict. They also help prevent the kidneys from retaining sodium and water. The acronym ACE stands for *angiotensin converting enzyme.*

Both short-acting (taken several times a day) and long-acting (typically taken once a day) ACE inhibitors are available for treatment of high blood pressure. ACE inhibitors are often prescribed for individuals with diabetes or heart failure because they may also benefit those conditions.

✔ **Angiotensin-receptor blockers (ARBs):** These drugs prevent the hormone angiotensin II from constricting the blood vessels and also causing the body to retain water and sodium. They target a different part of the renin-adrenergic system than ACE inhibitors or renin inhibitors (see next item on this list). These drugs have grown in popularity because many people tolerate them well without side effects. They also produce some benefits for people with diabetes and/or heart failure.

✔ **Direct renin inhibitors:** This is a very new class of drugs that's still being studied. These drugs block *renin,* the enzyme that regulates angiotensin II levels. The potential advantage of this class of drugs is that these drugs may reduce the fluctuation of blood pressure levels during the day.

✔ **Calcium channel blockers:** Also called *calcium antagonists,* calcium channel blockers inhibit the inward flow of calcium into cardiac and blood vessel tissues, thereby reducing the strength of heart contractions and the constriction of blood vessels.

✔ **Direct vasodilators:** These drugs are typically used in emergencies and act directly and quickly on the walls of the arteries and cause them to relax, thereby reducing the amount of pressure needed to pump blood through the arteries.

✔ **Combination medicines:** As I mention earlier, the majority of people require two medicines to control their high blood pressure. Obtaining those medications in a combined form often is possible and makes taking them simpler. If you're taking two or more medications for hypertension, ask your doctor whether a combination medicine is right for you.

Using drug treatment for cholesterol problems

In some instances, managing high LDL cholesterol or total cholesterol requires lipid-lowering medications in addition to lifestyle measures. This requirement is of particular necessity if

✔ Your blood cholesterol is extremely high

✔ You experience other major risk factors for heart disease

✔ You already have established CHD

In these instances, your physician probably will recommend drug therapy, in addition to lifestyle measures, to lower elevated blood cholesterol.

Classifying medications used to treat high cholesterol

Although a bewildering variety of cholesterol medications are available, the major ones fall into one of these four categories:

✔ **Statins:** Numerous statin medications help lower blood cholesterol. All of them act on an enzyme that is essential for the body to produce cholesterol. The statins slow down, or inhibit, this enzyme, which is called *HMG-CoA reductase.* (Remember that tongue twister, and you'll probably be one up on your doctor!) Many studies show that these medications powerfully reduce cholesterol and lower the risk of CHD. Statin medicines are particularly useful in lowering high levels of LDL cholesterol. Some individuals experience side effects with statins, including muscle and joint pain and muscle weakness. Always let your doctor know immediately about side effects. There are many different statins, and you and your doctor may be able to find one that works for you without side effects or your doctor may use another type of medication. Statins are the number one choice for treating elevated cholesterol levels in the blood.

✔ **Bile acid sequestrants:** These medications lower blood cholesterol by binding with cholesterol-containing bile acids in the intestines, from which they are later eliminated in the stool. Bile acid sequestrants have a long history of safe and effective use for lowering blood cholesterol. These medications are particularly valuable if you have elevated LDL cholesterol.

✔ **Fibric acids:** Fibric acids are particularly effective in lowering triglycerides, and they've demonstrated the ability to modestly lower LDL cholesterol. Fibric acids are particularly appropriate if you have high triglyceride levels and elevated LDL cholesterol. Tests also show that some of these medications raise HDL cholesterol — the good guys.

✔ **Nicotinic acid:** Nicotinic acid, which is a form of the B vitamin called niacin, is effective in lowering triglycerides and total blood cholesterol and in raising HDL cholesterol. Despite these benefits, some people may have difficulty tolerating this medication because of its side effects, which include itching and flushing of the skin and gastrointestinal distress.

Although niacin is inexpensive and available over the counter, never self-medicate for cholesterol control, because a physician must monitor you for major dangerous side effects.

Following up after beginning drug therapy

If your physician starts you on medication to help lower cholesterol, having your cholesterol level tested in four to six weeks after beginning the therapy is important. If adequate blood cholesterol lowering isn't achieved, increasing the dosage or adding a second medication may be necessary. Remember, lipid-lowering medications should always be used in conjunction with positive lifestyle measures, such as proper nutrition, increased physical activity, and weight management, if you're overweight.

Connecting with diabetes treatments

People who have diabetes are two to four times more likely to die of heart disease than people who don't have diabetes. It's also important to remember than people who have diabetes often have other risk factors for heart disease, particularly including high blood pressure, cholesterol problems, and obesity. So it is very important to keep diabetes under control (see Chapter 3 for some suggestions). If you are not able to control type 2 diabetes through lifestyle modification, including regular physical activity and an appropriate diet, then there are a number of oral medications that your doctor can choose from to help.

The recommended first-line drug for many individuals is metformin, particularly for people with diabetes who are also overweight. Metformin also appears to have a good effect on lipid levels, which also play a role in heart disease. Depending on your individual health conditions, your doctor may choose to use another oral anti-diabetic drug either in conjunction with metformin or instead of it. Progression to more severe type 2 diabetes may eventually require insulin replacement therapy.

Because people with diabetes so often have high blood pressure and cholesterol problems, the treatment protocol will also often include medications for these conditions. If this describes your situation, then your doctor will carefully monitor and balance all your medications. If you see more than one doctor for these conditions, be sure to always take a list of your current medications and the dosage to share whenever you see each of your doctors.

Treating Angina

If you have been diagnosed with stable angina (chest pain) that results from underlying coronary heart disease, your doctor will prescribe appropriate lifestyle measures to help you manage the condition and any risk factors. If you have angina, it's likely you also have cholesterol problems and elevated blood pressure and perhaps other risk factors. So you may already be taking medications for those conditions; if not, your doctor will probably prescribe appropriate medications to help you bring these conditions under control.

The goal in treating stable angina is to decrease the work of the heart, relax the coronary arteries so that more oxygenated blood reaches the heart, and decrease the tendency of blood to clot at the sites of fatty plaques. In many cases, aggressive treatment of the factors contributing to narrowing of coronary arteries can help you live comfortably and fully with the condition for many years. Some individuals following the regimen of rigorous lifestyle measures and appropriate medications have even experienced some regression of coronary artery disease.

Using medications to manage angina

As you can see in the following list, some of the medications prescribed to manage blood pressure and cholesterol are also used in treating angina. There are also additional important medications prescribed for the symptoms of angina. The following list highlights the roles of these common medications:

- **Nitrates:** Nitrates, particularly nitroglycerin, are valuable mainstays for treatment of angina. They relieve pressure on the heart and may also increase blood flow to the heart by causing the coronary arteries to dilate. Nitroglycerin often relieves discomfort quickly. Nitroglycerin/ nitrates may come in the form of tablets or sprays that you put under the tongue, a pill that you take by mouth, a cream that you apply to your skin, or a patch that you wear on your skin. Some people may experience headache as a side effect.

- **Beta blockers:** These medications, another mainstay of treatment, decrease how hard the heart must work by lowering blood pressure and decreasing heart rate. (For more on how beta blockers work, refer to the earlier section "Lowering high blood pressure.")

- **Calcium channel blockers (also called *calcium antagonists*):** This class of medicines blocks calcium flow into the muscle cells of arteries and enables arteries to dilate. They typically are less effective than nitrates and beta blockers in angina treatment; however, calcium antagonists may be used in conjunction with them. Calcium antagonists are particularly useful when any significant degree of spasm of the coronary arteries is present.

- **ACE inhibitors:** These drugs also help to relax or widen the blood vessels. They appear to be particularly helpful to people who have microvascular disease (narrowings of the small arteries of the heart, not the large arteries; go to Chapter 2 for more on MVD) or diabetes.

- **Ranolazine:** This relatively new anti-ischemic medication is used to help relax coronary blood vessels. Unlike some other drugs, however, it does not affect heart rate or blood pressure. It is usually prescribed with other drugs such as nitroglycerin or beta blockers.

- **Aspirin:** That's right, good old aspirin. Many people know that aspirin can relieve minor pain or fever, but they don't know that aspirin is important in treating angina because it helps prevent platelets from sticking to the walls of blood vessels and thereby contributing to any blood clot that may narrow or block off a coronary artery. Aspirin needs to be part of therapy for individuals with known or suspected CHD who haven't experienced any problems with bleeding.

  Research and experience show that using enteric, or coated, aspirin, which dissolves in the intestine, often helps lessen potential stomach irritation in some individuals who are sensitive to aspirin.

- **Anticoagulants and antiplatelet drugs:** The purpose of these drugs is to prevent clots on plaques from forming and prevent platelets from sticking together and contributing to clots. The goal is to prevent a heart attack. Some of these drugs may be used with aspirin to manage stable angina; others may be administered in the hospital to help in the acute setting of unstable angina. These drugs are also used to prevent strokes in people with an irregular heart rhythm, known as *atrial fibrillation*.

Benefiting from other medical therapies

Depending on the severity of your angina and your personal circumstances, your physician may recommend one or more of these other resources to help you manage your angina.

Cardiac rehabilitation

A good cardiac rehabilitation program (see more in Chapter 15) can help you learn to manage your angina and give you confidence to make lifestyle changes effectively and safely. Supervised by healthcare professionals, you can follow an individual physical activity program that will enable you to build strength, endurance, and fitness for your heart and muscles. Most rehab programs also offer dietary counseling, training in stress management, and other resources to help you succeed.

Extended external counterpulsion therapy (EECP)

Some individuals can benefit from this procedure in which large cuffs (similar to blood pressure cuffs) are fitted on the legs; they are then inflated and deflated in sync with the heart beat. This treatment can improve the flow of oxygen-rich blood to help relieve angina for some people. The typical course of treatment is 35 one-hour sessions over 7 weeks. It is usually prescribed when medication or other procedures have not sufficiently relieved angina symptoms.

Quitting smoking

This is one of the most important lifestyle changes that smokers with angina can make. I've put it as a separate therapy because you may wish to consult your physician about joining a support group and/or using medication to enhance your success in achieving this goal. For a detailed plan to help you give up cigarettes, refer to Chapter 11.

Recognizing when unstable angina is an emergency

If you are experiencing chest pain for this first time or if the symptoms of your stable angina change (pain doesn't resolve with rest, happens when you are asleep, increases in severity, and so on), then you must treat this as an emergency. Go directly to the emergency room.

Treating a Heart Attack Medically

When a heart attack occurs (see Chapter 2), the primary objectives of treatment are to act as fast as possible to save your life and to limit, even prevent, damage to the heart muscle. That's why it's crucial that you (or someone with you) call 911 to get medical help as quickly as possible. First responders are trained to take important first steps in treating a potential heart attack. Then healthcare teams at the emergency room and hospital will take over. In this section, I take you through the treatment protocol you can expect after you first experience the symptoms of a heart attack. Note that your own actions are the vital first steps.

Diagnosing and starting treatment for a potential heart attack

When you experience symptoms of a heart attack, call 911. Then, if you have nitroglycerine to treat angina, place one nitroglycerin pill under your tongue every five minutes. You can take up to three nitroglycerine pills. If you don't have nitroglycerine, take two aspirin and chew and swallow them.

Upon their arrival, emergency technicians will administer oxygen, give you aspirin and or nitroglycerin to improve blood flow (if you haven't already taken these), take an electrocardiogram, and start an intravenous line to deliver medicines. In many cases, particularly if you are not close to a hospital, they may start clot-busting medicines.

Receiving treatment in the emergency room

When you arrive at the emergency room, medical teams take immediate steps to determine whether you are having an acute heart attack and, if you are, to begin treatment. Here are some of the steps they'll take:

✔ Ask you questions about the nature of your symptoms and perform an electrocardiogram (ECG).

✔ If the ECG shows the characteristic patterns associated with acute heart attack, the team may administer clot-busting medications (antithrombolytics) to lessen the blockage and/or take you to the catheterization lab to perform angioplasty to treat the clot (see Chapter 13 for more on this surgical treatment).

✔ Draw blood (simultaneously with the ECG and physical examination) to be sent to the laboratory to check for chemical markers that indicate damage to the heart.

The development of increasingly sensitive blood tests for such biomarkers as cardiac troponin and the MB fraction of creatine kinase (CK-MB) that occur in the presence of acute injury to heart muscle cells has enabled more precise treatment for individual patients. These tests can detect much smaller areas of injury than imaging techniques.

✔ Possibly make use of a defibrillator to administer electric current to restore (or shock) the heart back into a normal rhythm.

✔ Continually ask you about the level of chest discomfort you may be experiencing. Always answer as accurately as you can. (A heart attack is no time for silent bravery!)

✔ Administer medicines to diminish your discomfort and start treatment. These medicines include aspirin to decrease the clotting ability of platelets and beta blockers to slow the heart rate and lower your blood pressure. These medications have been proven to decrease complications of acute heart attack.

All these procedures take place in rapid succession, with trained professionals calmly caring for you and reassuring you. Their goal is to create a calm atmosphere to diminish your anxiety.

Continuing treatment in the coronary care unit

If you're diagnosed with an acute heart attack, you're admitted to a specialized unit within the hospital called a *coronary care unit* (CCU). The CCU has specialized equipment and specially trained staff members who are able to continue your treatment and diagnose and quickly treat any complications that may occur from the acute heart attack. Your treatment typically contains a number of these elements:

- ✔ Continuing medical treatment to stabilize your condition, limit damage, and prevent complications.

- ✔ Continuous monitoring for potential complications such as heart rhythm problems, falling blood pressure, heart valve problems, continuing chest pain, or any other symptoms.

- ✔ Additional testing to confirm or rule out the diagnosis of acute heart attack and to determine the location and extent of the blockage. Testing also assesses the extent of injury to the heart muscle and the heart's ability to pump blood efficiently *(left ventricular function)*.

Depending on the outcome of these procedures and tests, further procedures like angioplasty or coronary artery bypass surgery (see Chapter 13) may be performed to restore or maximize blood flow to the heart muscle and minimize the amount of muscle that is damaged or dies.

Any or all of the treatment measures described in the sections that follow often are used to treat the early stages of a heart attack.

Preventing additional blood clots

Additional blood clots are a dangerous possibility for people who have just had a heart attack. The following medications help prevent more blood clots from occurring:

- ✔ **Aspirin** is used to decrease the "stickiness" of platelets and thus lessen their ability to continue to form blood clots within the coronary arteries.

- ✔ **Anticoagulants,** or blood thinners, also protect against the tendency of additional blood clots forming either in the coronary arteries or within one of the heart's chambers near the damaged area of muscle.

- ✔ **Platelet receptor inhibitors** act in conjunction with aspirin to further keep platelets from sticking together.

- ✔ **Other medications** may be part of your treatment. If you have elevated cholesterol or high blood pressure, you may be given additional medications to treat these conditions. (See Chapter 9 for more about cholesterol and Chapter 8 for more about high blood pressure.)

Controlling cardiac pain

Pain management is important in treating an acute heart attack, because cardiac pain is a marker for continued damage to the fragile cells of the heart muscle. Controlling pain indicates decreasing damage. Pain management typically is accomplished with a combination of medicines such as pain relievers, nitrates, and beta blockers:

- ✔ **Pain relievers,** also called *analgesics,* can be used during the acute phase of a heart attack. Morphine is probably the most commonly used.

- ✔ **Nitrates,** such as nitroglycerin, increase blood flow through coronary arteries and decrease the work of the heart.

- ✔ **Beta blockers** decrease pressure on the heart and slow the heart rate, both of which decrease the demand from the heart muscle for oxygen.

- ✔ **Oxygen** improves the supply of oxygenated blood to the heart muscle. This is typically delivered through an oxygen mask or an oxygen tube that's placed in the nose.

Continuing monitoring and testing

In the CCU, monitoring is continuous. Additional tests such as electrocardiograms, physical examinations, and echocardiograms are given at regular intervals to look for any complications. (For more about common heart tests, see Chapter 22.)

Recuperating from a heart attack

After you've been stabilized and the acute events surrounding your heart attack have been treated, you enter what most large hospitals call a step-down unit. Your stay in the step-down unit will be for several days, typically until you can begin rehabilitation from the heart attack.

The rehabilitation process starts in the hospital and takes place during the next few months after you're discharged from the hospital. The rehabilitative steps that you take in the hospital include

- ✔ Changing over to medications that can be taken orally.

- ✔ Working with your physician and trained cardiac rehabilitation specialists to assess your condition and start treatment of risk factors for heart disease that may be present. (Yes, it's back to school for you.)

- ✔ Beginning a progressive increase in physical activity, starting with slow walking initially in your room, followed by walking in the hospital hallway. After you leave the hospital, you will typically continue in an outpatient rehabilitation program.

Potentially repairing damaged heart muscle

In recent years, quick medical response to heart attacks and increasingly effective medical and surgical treatments have done much to decrease damage to the heart muscle for many patients. The ideal treatment, however, would be to be able to actually reverse the damage and to enable regeneration of healthy heart muscle. Currently, a number of different streams of research are examining innovative methods for possible regeneration therapy such as activating or inducing various types of stem cells or activating some of the heart's own potential regenerative properties. No approach has been approved for use yet, but these are promising avenues of research.

In addition to the physical and medical issues, almost every patient undergoes a spectrum of emotional responses to acute heart attack. These responses vary from extreme anxiety during the actual event to depression and remorse afterward. The good news: The vast majority of individuals who survive a heart attack go on to lead long and productive lives. The process of cardiac rehabilitation is so important that I devote Chapter 15 to this topic.

Managing Heart Failure

Heart failure occurs when the heart no longer adequately pumps blood to the lungs and throughout the body. Many conditions including heart attack and underlying conditions can cause the heart muscle to try to compensate by enlarging, thickening, or beating faster.

Treatments for heart failure generally attempt to counteract the negative effects of the heart's own compensatory mechanisms or to strengthen the pumping ability of a weakened or damaged heart directly. These treatments range from lifestyle modifications to a variety of medicines and procedures.

Some of the treatment programs that you can undergo or that your doctor will institute to help treat heart failure are described in this section.

Modifying your lifestyle

Modifying certain lifestyle practices, as your doctor may direct, can help treat congestive heart failure and enhance the comfort and quality of your life as you live with the condition. Here are some common modifications.

✔ Weighing yourself daily to check for rapid weight gain that usually indicates fluid retention.

✔ Restricting sodium because it causes your body to retain fluids. If you have heart failure, even a small increase in your sodium level can tip you over into a very serious bout of lung congestion.

✔ Limiting fluid and alcohol consumption. Alcohol further depresses the pumping ability of the heart, and increased fluids can raise the fluid buildup in the lungs and the rest of the body.

✔ Performing light to moderate physical activity to help the heart pump more efficiently and other muscles work more efficiently. More efficient pumping and working reduces demands on the heart. Of course, if you experience heart failure, you won't be training for a marathon or triathlon — easy does it. Very carefully, too.

Before undertaking any exercise program, you absolutely must talk to your doctor about the amount and best type of exercise for you and the warning signs of over-exercising. Many cardiac rehab programs have special protocols for patients with heart failure, including customized exercise programs.

✔ Stopping smoking. Your physician will urge you to make quitting your first priority. Smoking not only contributes to the underlying causes of heart failure but also has a direct effect on heart rate and blood pressure. (See Chapter 11 to find strategies for quitting smoking.)

Treating heart failure with medications

A variety of medicines are useful in treating heart failure. Not all of these drugs are right for all patients, and combinations of drugs often are used to address individual situations. Here are some of the medicines that your physician may use:

✔ **Diuretics:** Often called *fluid pills* or *water pills* by the people who take them, diuretics help reduce the amount of fluid in the body and are useful in individuals who are experiencing heart failure and fluid retention. As I discuss in Chapter 8, diuretics also are useful in treating hypertension.

✔ **Digitalis:** Digitalis (or digoxin) helps the heart contract more vigorously. Digitalis was one of the first medicines to be used for treating heart failure, and it continues to be one of the best medicines for stimulating the heart to pump more effectively and for reducing the symptoms of heart failure. (Digitalis was initially was made from the foxglove plant — Latin name *digitalis*. Deposit that in your trivia bank!) Because of the newer drugs listed below, digitalis has become second or even third line therapy for heart failure.

✔ **ACE inhibitors:** Although originally developed for treating high blood pressure, ACE inhibitors can reduce the work of the heart by decreasing the amount of pressure in blood vessels against which the heart must pump. Studies indicate this effect may slow losses in the heart's pumping ability and improve the quality of life and survival in people with heart failure.

Although ace inhibitors have become an important part of first line therapy for heart failure, several studies now show that many physicians underuse them. Feel free to ask your physician more about them.

✔ **Angiotensin II receptor blockers (ARBs):** Your physician may choose to use ARBs in place of or, in some cases, in conjunction with ACE inhibitors. Research also shows that they may be useful for individuals who cannot take ACE inhibitors or beta blockers (see the next item in this list).

✔ **Beta blockers:** Beta blockers (another drug developed to treat hypertension) slow the heart's contraction rate, thus reducing its pumping action. Certain beta blockers may be valuable to some patients with heart failure because they reduce the likelihood that these patients will suffer significant heart rhythm problems.

Severe heart failure may also be treated by drugs that cause the heart to beat more strongly (isotropic therapy) and by implantable pace makers or defibrillators, depending on the individual patient's symptoms.

Treating Arrhythmias

Day in and day out, the beat goes on — the heartbeat, that is — and all that beating depends on the heart's electrical system. When this electrical system suffers from some insult, such as lack of blood flow to the heart, it can cause cardiac rhythm problems, called *arrhythmias.*

There are many different types of arrhythmias with different causes and therefore many different treatments. These include lifestyle measures, medications, and medical procedures such as *cardioversion* (defibrillation) and implantable pacemakers and defibrillators.

Using lifestyle measures

Palpitations, the most common *symptom* of arrhythmia, may be caused by or made worse by practices such as drinking too many caffeinated beverages (coffee, tea, and many soft drinks), consuming too much alcohol, not effectively treating stress, or not obtaining adequate rest. Changing any or all of these lifestyle measures often can make palpitations disappear as they ease the underlying problem.

Prescribing medications

A bewildering variety of medications are available to treat cardiac arrhythmias. Likewise, the manner by which these medications are administered can be very complex. So if you have a serious rhythm problem, your personal physician probably will consult with a cardiologist who is skilled in the use of these medications.

There are too many medications and their uses are too complex to describe here. However, as an example, consider medications for *atrial fibrillation*, the most common type of problem. In "A-fib," one or both of the upper chambers of the heart may beat irregularly, contracting very fast and not fully. This causes blood to pool in the atria and increases the risk of blood clots, which in turn increases the risk of heart attack and stroke. So your physician will typically prescribe clot prevention medications, also called blood thinners, such as warfarin, aspirin, or one of the newer medications. Medical therapy also aims to slow down the heart rate and help return it to normal by using such medications as beta blockers, calcium channel blockers, digitalis, or other medications. Some people with A-fib may also need medications to control rhythm; these may be started in the hospital and are always monitored very carefully because the medications can cause other serious problems.

As the preceding example shows, controlling atrial fibrillation and other rhythm problems is not "take a pill and forget it." If you have heart rhythm problems, work closely with your doctor and report any difficulties or changes in symptoms.

Employing electrical therapy

In many cases, arrhythmias are treated with techniques and devices that use electricity to manage the heart's electrical system.

Cardioversion

You can describe this form of treatment by saying it takes one to fix one. Because the heart is an electrical system, the skilled application of an external source of electricity can jolt the heart back into its normal rhythm. This process is called *cardioversion*.

During cardioversion therapy, the patient usually is sedated and put to sleep (of course, in an emergency, time is not taken for sedation). Two electrical paddles are applied to the chest wall at the level of the heart, and an electrical current is passed through the heart. This shock causes the electrical system to reboot itself and often pop back into the normal sinus rhythm that is desirable.

Cardioversion can effectively treat various cardiac arrhythmias, including atrial fibrillation, atrial flutter, ventricular tachycardia, and ventricular fibrillation. Cardioversion, also called *defibrillation,* is literally a lifesaver in emergencies when acute ventricular tachycardia and ventricular fibrillation threaten immediate death because the heart is not putting out any oxygenated blood. Modern cardioversion or defibrillation equipment is capable of sensing underlying cardiac rhythm and applying exactly the right amount of shock at exactly the right time to maximize the likelihood of converting the heart back into its normal rhythm.

Automatic implantable defibrillators

Automatic implantable defibrillators, also known as implantable cardioverter-defibrillators (ICDs), perform a particularly effective type of cardioversion, and their development has provided new leases on life to patients with serious ventricular rhythm problems. When implanted inside the chest, the device monitors the heart's rhythm and quickly administers an electrical shock as needed to correct any serious arrhythmias. Although when the defibrillator goes off, or fires, patients feel a sensation as if they've been kicked in the chest, they typically don't mind receiving that kind of wakeup call. They say it's certainly preferable to the alternative.

Pacemaker therapy

Pacemakers typically are used when the heart has very slow rhythm. Modern cardiac pacemakers can sequentially pace the atria and the ventricles to generate an effective cardiac output. These pacemakers are able to sense the heart's own rhythm and kick into action only when that rhythm slows to a certain point. Advances in electronic design and battery power also have enabled pacemakers to be made smaller and last for many years between battery changes. And, to the delight of those who rely on them, modern pacemakers are not sensitive to microwave ovens and the like.

Treating Valve Problems

At this time, there is no medication that treats heart valve disease. Severe valve problems are treated with various surgical options, including repair and replacement. Other heart problems that could make valve problems worse, such as high blood pressure or atrial fibrillation, are typically treated by medications and lifestyle measures. If a valve repair or replacement, such as using a mechanical valve, increases the risk of blood clots forming, then anticlotting medication is usually part of the treatment protocol.

Keeping Track of Your Medications

As this chapter shows, there are many, many medications used in treating various forms of heart disease. Also, many people, particularly as they reach middle age and beyond, may have more than one form of heart disease and therefore take a variety of medications.

One of the most important things you can do to work with your doctors is to keep an up-to-date list of all your medications. That's every last medication you take for any condition — whether they are prescription medications or over-the-counter drugs and supplements. Most people today have more than one doctor. Making sure that all your medications work well together and don't have potentially negative interactions is an ongoing challenge.

So here's what to do. Open a spreadsheet or text document on your computer. (If you don't have one, hand print the list on a piece of paper that can be photocopied.) List the following:

- ✔ Name of the medication (example, metoprolol succinate ER)
- ✔ The size of the dose (example, 50 mg)
- ✔ How often you take it (example, 1/day)
- ✔ Any other special instruction

Keep the list up to date. Print out a copy and take it to each doctor's visit.

Chapter 13

The 411 on Invasive and Surgical Procedures

*A*lthough many people with heart disease manage their conditions with lifestyle modifications and drug therapy, many other problems ranging from blocked coronary arteries to heart valve failures require minimally invasive medical procedures or surgery to restore higher heart function and quality of life for the patient. In this chapter, I discuss medical and surgical procedures commonly used to treat atherosclerotic narrowing and blockage of coronary arteries, heart valve problems, and rhythm problems.

Understanding Percutaneous Coronary Interventions (PCIs)

When atherosclerosis severely narrows or blocks any of the major coronary arteries, threatening to cause a heart attack, *percutaneous coronary interventions,* or *PCIs,* often are used to relieve the problem. That fancy word *percutaneous* simply means that the cardiologist performs the procedure through the skin. (Don't you love medspeak?)

Most such procedures use a catheter that is inserted into the blocked vessel. Various devices and techniques help the surgical team see exactly what is going on in a blocked artery:

✔ A *fluoroscope,* which delivers real-time X-ray pictures of the vessel and catheter movements to a screen, enables the cardiologist and medical-care team to view exactly what's happening as it happens.

✔ Intravascular ultrasound may be used to enable the doctor to determine the size of the interior of the blocked artery, which helps determine what size catheter balloons and stents to use.

✔ Using fractional flow reserve assessment may help the doctor decide how severe the blockage is by assessing restriction to the blood flow through the artery.

PCIs typically take place in cardiac catheterization labs. Patient preparation and recovery are similar for most procedures. Before the procedure, patients usually receive a sedative to relax them, anticoagulants to prevent potentially dangerous blood clots forming around the catheter or instruments during the procedure, and other medications as needed. Local anesthesia numbs the area where the catheter is inserted, usually in the femoral artery in the upper thigh but sometimes in the arm. After the procedure is finished, the patient remains in recovery until the catheter sheath is removed from the insertion site and there's no chance of bleeding or complication at that site. Patients may then either remain in the hospital or go home the same day, depending on the individual patient's condition, the nature of the procedure, and the technique used for ensuring that the catheter insertion site in the artery won't bleed. If you need one of the following PCI procedures, your doctor gives you complete instructions.

Opening blocked arteries with coronary angioplasty

Coronary angioplasty, also called *balloon angioplasty,* is a minimally invasive procedure that can quickly restore or improve blood flow through blocked arteries in patients for whom the procedure is appropriate. More than a half million patients benefit from angioplasty every year. Its formal name, which you may hear from your cardiologist or find in patient information, is *percutaneous transluminal coronary angioplasty* (PTCA).

Using the technique of heart catheterization, the cardiologist moves a specialized catheter equipped with a high-pressure balloon (on its tip) into the narrowed or blocked coronary artery or arteries. Once the catheter enters the narrowed section of the artery, the balloon is inflated. The inflated balloon stretches the artery and literally compresses the plaque up against the side of the blood vessel (see Figure 13-1). This procedure opens up the artery, enabling greater blood flow.

One drawback of conventional angioplasty is that in 25 percent to 50 percent of cases, the narrowing recurs in the artery, an event called *restenosis.* That is why medicine-eluting *stents* (devices that support the expanded walls of the treated arteries) are almost always used in PCI today.

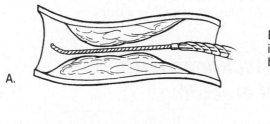

A.

Balloon catheter inserted into artery at blockage by plaques.

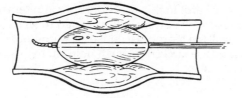

B.

Balloon inflated.

Figure 13-1:
Balloon
angioplasty.

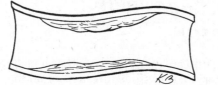

C.

Plaques reduced following angioplasty.

Illustration by Kathryn Born

Holding arteries open with coronary stenting

In most angioplasties today, the cardiologist places a device called a stent in the area where the angioplasty has occurred. These mechanical devices look a little like coiled springs and are designed to hold blood vessels open.

Stents significantly lessen the chance that the narrowing will recur, but they don't completely prevent it. Therefore, using the new generation of specialized stents called *drug-eluting stents,* which incorporate a time-release drug, is usual to provide additional protection against renarrowing.

In the few cases where restenosis occurs with drug-eluting stents, it usually occurs because tissue from the artery's lining has grown through the mesh of the stent, rather than from regrowth of atherosclerotic plaque. A very new type of imaging called *opticalcoherence tomography (OCT)* appears to provide a higher resolution image than intra-arterial ultrasound and enables cardiologists to look closely at individual areas of a stent to better understand the type of restenosis. OCT is also delivered by a catheter.

Removing blockages with coronary atherectomy

Coronary atherectomy may be the procedure of choice when the fatty plaque blocking the artery is very hard. In this procedure, a catheter tipped with a tiny metal cone equipped with cutting edges is used to shave away the plaque from the artery walls in a process similar to Roto-Rootering. The loosened plaque particles then are sucked through holes in the catheter tip and removed from the blood vessel.

Removing blockages with laser angioplasty

Laser angioplasty is similar to an atherectomy in that it also removes the plaque narrowing the artery. In this procedure, a laser on the end of the catheter is used to incinerate the fatty plaque deposits.

Preventing renarrowing with brachytherapy

Coronary brachytherapy is another technique that cardiologists may consider using for individuals who have experienced a renarrowing or blockage of a stented artery. In appropriate cases, the blockage is caused by overgrowth of endothelial tissue lining the artery, not clot formation.

This procedure uses a special catheter placed inside the artery to deliver a small dose of beta or gamma radiation directly to the artery lining where the blockage is located. Although the procedure appears beneficial in the short-term, it does have significant side effects and the long-term effectiveness of the procedure is not yet known. At present, cardiologists are using this technique for only a few patients who have severe problems.

Using angioplasty immediately after a heart attack

In certain cases immediately after an individual has had a heart attack and where the conditions are appropriate, the cardiologist may use one of the forms of angioplasty I've just discussed to remove the clot (thrombus) that caused the heart attack and/or to widen the blocked artery. The objective is to restore blood flow to the damaged part of the heart muscle as quickly as possible and thus preserve as much function as possible. This procedure can be lifesaving in many cases.

Looking at Coronary Bypass Surgery

Certain problems with severely blocked arteries may require coronary bypass surgery. In addition to conventional *coronary artery bypass grafting* (CABG — often pronounced "cabbage" in the lingo of physicians), recent research has developed several types of less invasive coronary bypass surgery that appear to offer equally effective results and shorter recovery times for selected individuals. Such surgery is performed by cardiac surgeons, who train first as general surgeons and then specialize in cardiac surgery. Although they belong to different specialties, cardiologists and cardiac surgeons work closely together. Here's a look at the "gold standard" CABG and new less-invasive bypass surgical procedures.

Understanding coronary artery bypass grafting

In coronary artery bypass grafting, a piece of artery or vein is used to bypass the blockage in a coronary artery and restore blood flow.

In the conventional form of CABG, an incision is made through the breastbone (sternum) and the chest is opened to reach the heart (hence the term *open-heart surgery*). The donor vessels for the bypass grafts are also prepared; they come from the patient's own body. Usually, the left interior mammary artery in the chest is used to bypass blockage in the left anterior descending artery on the front of the heart. The other grafts may come from other arteries or saphenous veins from the legs.

In most cases, the patient also is placed on a heart-lung machine (or pump oxygenator) that takes over for the heart, which then is stopped for the surgery. Where possible with an arterial graft vessel, the surgeon usually leaves one end attached to the artery's blood source and secures the other end to the blocked coronary artery below the blockage (or *occlusion*). Some artery graphs and all venous graphs are typically attached to the aorta on one end and below the blockage at the other end thereby allowing blood to flow again in the previously blocked artery. The surgeon decides which graft vessels (arteries or veins) and procedures to use, based on the location of the blockage, the size of the blockage, and the size of the patient's coronary arteries.

When all the grafts to be performed are complete, the patient is removed from the heart-lung machine, and the heart is restarted. The breastbone is rejoined using surgical wires that remain permanently in place after stabilizing the breastbone and aiding in its healing. After the surgery is complete, CABG patients are carefully monitored in the Intensive Cardiac Care Unit (ICCU).

Bypassing blocked coronary arteries with less invasive surgery

Conventional bypass surgery is major surgery. It's about as *major* as surgery can get. The breastbone must be split, the heart stopped, and the patient's life supported by a heart-lung machine for several hours. This surgery has a highly successful track record, but its risks and complexity offer potential for complications for many patients. Full recovery also takes about three to six months for most patients. As a result, cardiac surgeons and specialists constantly are working to develop surgical techniques that are less difficult and less risky but still produce quality outcomes for patients.

Currently, there are several less-invasive procedures are being used in selected, appropriate cases.

Minimally invasive direct coronary artery bypass (MIDCAB)

Unlike conventional CABG, in which the breastbone is split to open the chest and provide access to the heart, in MIDCAB, the cardiac surgeon works with special instruments through a small keyhole incision in the chest wall that's about 2.5 inches to 4 inches (6 cm to 10 cm) across. As part of the incision, a tiny piece of costal cartilage on the front of a rib is removed to provide access. On most patients, the surgeon can perform the bypass without placing the patient on a heart-lung machine.

This procedure is typically used only in selected patients who need only one or two bypasses on the front of the heart. In some heart centers, the surgeon may also use robot-assisted techniques.

Off-pump coronary artery bypass (OPCAB)

This technique enables surgeons to stabilize a beating heart to safely perform surgery on it. To perform OPCAB, the surgeon makes the same type and size incision through the breastbone as for conventional bypass surgery. Then, instead of placing the patient on a heart-lung machine, the surgeon uses a sta-bilizing device that immobilizes small sections of the heart where the surgeon is working while allowing the heart to keep beating.

Potential benefits from OPCAB include decreased blood transfusions, decreased risk of stroke, and fewer problems with lungs, kidneys, and mental clarity, and possibly quicker recovery times. To date, most longitudinal stud-ies have not shown any increase in longevity with this procedure compared to conventional CABG.

Hybrid coronary revascularization

This minimally invasive technique combines minimally invasive bypass sur-gery with coronary stenting. It is not widely available yet because research continues into whether it offers advantages over conventional or minimally invasive CABG.

Typically minimally invasive surgery is used to perform a graft of an internal mammary artery to a blockage in an artery on the front of the heart. Other blockages, usually just one or two, are treated with angioplasty and stenting.

Exploring Heart Valve Surgery

Injury or disease may cause heart valves to malfunction in two basic ways:

- ✔ **Stenosis:** Constricting or narrowing so that they do not let enough blood flow through
- ✔ **Regurgitation:** Leaking as the result of defects that prevent them from closing properly

Manifestations of both problems may require medical or surgical repair. Severe malfunctions may require valve replacement.

Opening narrowed valves with valvuloplasty

In *percutaneous balloon valvuloplasty*, the cardiologist inserts a catheter tipped with a high-pressure balloon through a blood vessel into the heart. After posi-tioning the balloon in the narrowed valve, the cardiologist inflates the balloon to stretch the constricted valve. The likelihood of the valve reconstricting is about 50 percent, so this procedure is used most commonly for individuals who have only mild or moderate valve narrowing or who cannot tolerate open-heart surgery. Newer minimally invasive surgical techniques are enabling more high-risk individuals to have longer-lasting repairs.

Repairing heart valves with surgery

For both narrowed and leaking heart valves, the conventional procedure for repair uses open-heart surgery and the heart-lung machine. In such a procedure, the surgeon cuts into the valve to surgically remodel its structures, enabling them to function properly. The restorative results of such surgery usually are long-lasting.

Today there are also minimally invasive techniques for use in valve surgery. This type of surgery still requires placing the patient on the heart-lung machine, but the surgeon accesses the heart through several small incisions rather than by cracking open the breast bone. The development of special instruments and a small video camera that allows the surgery team to view the heart and valve has made this type of surgery possible. Some such surgeries may also be robotically assisted, which enables great precision. The goal of minimally invasive surgery is to lower surgical risk and reduce recovery times.

Current research is actively exploring ways in which valve repair surgery may be performed without any incisions by working through a catheter. As in minimally invasive valve surgery, developing the right special tools and techniques are crucial to bringing this promising approach to fruition. A transcatheter procedure for replacing the aortic valve is already available (see the next section).

Replacing defective heart valves

When any of the four cardiac valves becomes so damaged that it cannot function properly and cannot be repaired surgically, the damaged valve needs to be replaced with one of the following types of prosthetic valves:

- **Mechanical valves,** which are constructed from metal and/or other synthetic materials
- **Natural valves,** which make use of human or animal tissue and come in three types:
  - **Xenograph,** a specially treated porcine valve from a pig or bovine valve from a cow
  - **Autograph,** a valve shaped from the patient's own tissue
  - **Homograph,** a human valve from a cadaver donor

Each of these different valves has particular advantages and disadvantages. Surgeons always discuss the pros and cons of each type of valve with their patients. As in coronary artery bypass surgery, valve replacement usually requires open-heart surgery and the use of a heart-lung machine.

One new minimally invasive technique, however, is available for selected high-risk patients. In this technique, the replacement valve is delivered via a catheter to the site of the aortic valve inside the heart. Then the compressed valve is opened up and fitted over the existing diseased valve. The new valve is then secured so that it functions in place of the diseased valve. The procedure is commonly known as *TAVR* (transcatheter aortic valve replacement) or *TAVI* (transcatheter aortic valve implantation.) At present this new procedure is used only for very high-risk patients who are unable to tolerate open-heart or minimally invasive surgery. That means that most people experiencing this procedure are in their 70s and 80s. To date, the outcomes of the procedure are very promising, but long-term evaluation has just begun.

Treating Rhythm Problems with the Electric Company

Because the complex electrical impulses that control the heart's rhythm and contraction are so critical, a whole branch of cardiology has grown to detect rhythm abnormalities and correct underlying electrical problems in the heart. In this section, I discuss the most commonly used medical or surgical electrical procedures involving the heart (see also Chapter 12 for drug therapies that address rhythm problems).

Cardioversion

This procedure applies a small amount of electrical current to the heart, using the same equipment that is used for defibrillation (explained in Chapter 12). Although the procedure is not invasive, for clarity I've grouped it with the rest of the electric company.

Cardioversion can be used to treat certain rhythm abnormalities, such as

- Irregular beating of the heart's atria, or booster pumps (*atrial fibrillation*)
- A rapid heartbeat originating in the booster pumps (*atrial tachycardia*)
- A rapid heartbeat originating in the ventricles (*ventricular tachycardia*)

Implantable cardioverter defibrillators (ICD)

Thanks to technological advances, tiny defibrillators about the size of a pacemaker can be implanted in the chest wall. Cardiologists increasingly are using these devices in individuals with serious arrhythmias who have survived episodes of sudden cardiac death or who are at high risk of cardiac collapse because of persistent ventricular arrhythmia or severe heart failure. The device monitors heart rhythms and automatically delivers an appropriate shock as necessary to restore proper rhythms. Newer devices function dually as both a ICD and pacemaker; in addition, they can record arrhythmic episodes and perform some electrophysiological testing, functions that allow your cardiologist to fine-tune your treatment.

Strong magnetic fields can affect how your implantable cardioverter defibrillator (ICD) functions. The American Heart Association notes that it's safe to use many household devices that have magnetic fields if you take some precautions:

✔ It's okay to use a microwave but don't work very long within 2 feet of an active microwave.

✔ Most household devices usually won't affect your ICD but to be safe keep 6 inches between your ICD and any device. For example, use your cellphone on the ear away from the side where your ICD is implanted. Store the phone in an opposite side pocket. Though they pose little risk, keeping a little distance (at least 6 inches) between your ICD implant and electronic devices also goes for a TV remote, MP3 player, earphones/buds or a tablet, laptop or desktop computer.

✔ Stay 2 feet away from electrical generators and light welding equipment.

✔ The American Heart Association also warns there are some devices you should avoid.

  • Don't use heavy duty (arc) welding equipment

  • Don't use magnetic mattress pads or pillows or other magnetic devices that you wear.

  • Don't use electronic body fat scales or ab stimulators

  • Stay 12 inches away from battery chargers, electric fences and the like

  • Always tell your doctors you have an ICD. If you must undergo some tests such as an MRI (magnetic resonance imaging) or other scans, your doctor will need to be aware of your ICD to make adjustments.

It's smart to carry a wallet card that notes that you have an ICD. Also always tell security personnel before security scans. It's okay to walk normally through a scanning device, but ask to be scanned if possible some other way than with a handheld scanner.

Pacemakers

Pacemakers are used, either temporarily or permanently, to speed up a heart that is beating too slowly, a condition called *bradycardia* (*brady* = slow; *cardia* = heartbeat). Pacemakers actually *pace* the heartbeat by delivering electrical impulses that are very similar to the heart's own electrical system. The typical pacemaker employed now has one electrical beat that goes into the atrium, and one that goes into the ventricle. These *A-V pacemakers* are powered by batteries that can last for many years.

Pacemakers typically are placed in the front of the chest using a minor surgical procedure to create a pocket under the skin. The electrodes then are threaded into the right atrium or ventricle or into both, depending upon the type of pacemaker.

Though there is little danger that electric and electronic devices will affect modern pacemakers, it doesn't hurt to be aware of your surroundings or follow the precautions for ICDs listed in the preceding section.

Cardiac electrophysiology

As the most advanced form of electrical work on the heart, electrophysiology takes place in specialized laboratories that resemble heart catheterization labs.

Specialized electrical catheters are placed into various portions of the heart, where either monitoring or corrective electrical work can be performed either to diagnose or correct rhythm problems or other electrical abnormalities. For example, to treat chronic tachycardia (fast heart rate) in carefully selected patients, the electrophysiologist may perform a procedure known as *ablation*, in which heat from catheter-delivered radio frequency energy is used precisely to destroy the tiny, selected parts of the heart's electrical system that are causing the tachycardia. Because they're so specialized, electrophysiology procedures typically are performed in large hospital centers.

Considering Other Forms of Cardiac Surgery

Cardiac surgeons also perform operations on other aspects of the heart, such as removing cardiac tumors, repairing congenital heart disease, and performing various pieces of surgery on the lungs. Should you need this type of surgery, your physician will explain what to expect and how to prepare for the surgery.

Chapter 14

Exploring Complementary Therapies

*Y*ou know by now that I believe you can do many things in your daily life to enhance your short- and long-term quality of life. But where do complementary and alternative therapies fit in?

Let me say right from the beginning that Western medicine doesn't have all the answers. Various therapeutic techniques, personal practices, and products that fall under the rubric of complementary or alternative medicine can be beneficial. But because the terms can be used to cover so many areas, the old warning of caveat emptor — let the buyer beware — certainly applies here. However, if you're careful and use *proven* complementary or alternative techniques judiciously and in combination with the many benefits of modern Western cardiovascular medicine, you can derive important benefits without taking unnecessary risks.

In this chapter, I look at some complementary or alternative therapies that have been proven to be beneficial in the fight against heart disease. I also discuss how to judge which techniques are questionable or even pure baloney.

Defining Complementary and Alternative Medicine

Complementary and alternative medicine typically describe healthcare approaches that originated outside mainstream Western or "conventional" medicine. In the last twenty years, as scientific studies have validated some of them, many of these approaches have become respected complements to what we might call "conventional" medicine. For example, guided imagery is now a mainstay in pain management.

Here are the key definitions to keep in mind:

- ✔ The term *complementary* describes such approaches that are used in conjunction with conventional techniques.
- ✔ The term *alternative*, in contrast, applies to approaches that are typically used instead or in place of mainstream medical approaches.

The difficulty with these nicely discreet definitions, of course, is that you may see them used higgledy-piggledy to represent a number of things in popular media and marketing and on the Internet.

As a cardiologist, I want the very best care that's effective for each individual patient I see. So I am glad to see that the National Center for Complementary and Alternative Medicine (NCCAM) points out that very few people use only alternative medicine. Most use complementary methods along with more conventional medical approaches. And the designation of specific techniques may well change over time as more and more well-designed, rigorous scientific studies test the more promising complementary and alternative therapies.

Complementary medicine has come to include a variety of behavioral techniques, such as relaxation methods or meditation and other spiritual techniques, in addition to a number of different clinical approaches, such as chiropractic, massage, and herbal remedies. As a practical matter, it has come to include both *mind therapy* (behavioral) and *body therapy* (clinical). Mind therapies include mental imagery, hypnosis, relaxation, and so on. Body therapies include not only chiropractic but also acupuncture and herbal treatments. In the following sections in this chapter, I discuss just a few of these more common approaches.

Recognizing the Difference between the Placebo Effect and Proof

Emotions tend to run pretty high when people talk about complementary or alternative medicine. Some people believe that the techniques of complementary or alternative medicine have made enormous differences in their lives. However, until recent years, few of these techniques had undergone rigorous scientific testing, so little scientific evidence has been available about whether many of these techniques are clinically effective. That situation is changing, but much research remains to be done. So doctors remain skeptical.

In a sense, both positions are right. Thanks to the complex interdependency of the human mind and body, you sometimes get benefits from a therapeutic action just because you believe you will. Physicians first observed this phenomenon while testing whether particular substances were biologically active. Part of a group of test subjects received a potential drug, and, for control, the other half received a pharmacologically inert substance called a *placebo* (often a sugar pill). None of the test subjects, however, knew exactly which substance they received. In any type of experiment, some subjects who were taking the placebo showed an improvement in symptoms. This response became known as the *placebo effect*.

The placebo effect is not phony or bad; it's just a fact of human psychology. Most people can, and often do, use it positively. Your admirable attachment to teddy bears is a case in point. What is a teddy bear? Objectively, it's just cloth pieced together and stuffed. Can a stuffed bear reach out and give you a hug? Can a teddy bear help you fend off the monsters of the night? Yet as children (and beyond), virtually everyone has drawn immense comfort from their teddies during times of stress or anxiety. On a more complex level, similar things are happening when people search for treatments for what ails them.

Western medicine tests potential medicines and therapies by conducting scientific trials designed to control for the placebo effect. Until only recently, few techniques or substances in complementary or alternative medicine were put through this type of controlled scientific trial. Although that doesn't mean some substances cannot have benefit, you nevertheless always need to sort through the evidence as best you can and educate yourself to determine which substances and techniques in complementary or alternative medicine have proven benefits.

Finding and understanding scientific information about various alternative therapies is a challenge, but the National Center for Complementary & Alternative Medicine (NCCAM), which is a branch of the National Institutes of Health, provides a number of excellent online resources, including links to Complementary and Alternative Medicine on PubMed and other databases, and tips on how you can conduct searches of alternative medicine subjects. You can consult the NCCAM Web site at `nccam.nih.gov`.

Drawing on Lifestyle Medicine and the Mind/Body Connection

If you look at various lists of complementary or alternative therapies from a variety of sources, you're likely to find the lifestyle practices that you probably think of as mainstream right at the top of the list — sound nutrition, appropriate physical activity and exercise, and stress reduction, for example. In fact, these once-alternative therapies have become mainstream medicine because a huge body of evidence proves that many daily habits and practices in these areas clearly lower your risk of heart disease and help you manage many heart conditions. At the same time, each of these proven lifestyle measures offers an *alternative* that often can render advanced cardiac techniques or medicines used in Western medicine unnecessary or can serve as a *complement* to such techniques.

Three areas of lifestyle medicine are so important that I've devoted a chapter to each: See Chapter 5 on nutrition and physical activity, Chapter 10 on weight management, and Chapter 6 on using the mind/body connection to reduce stress.

In this section, I discuss additional mind/body techniques that you may find useful in helping reduce your risk of heart disease or managing your heart disease to achieve the quality of life you desire.

Tapping into mind/body techniques

No other organ in the body, with the possible exception of the brain, is more affected by your emotional state than the heart. Profound mind/body connections impact everything from hypertension to cardiac rhythms. In addition to the techniques for stress reduction that I discuss in Chapter 6, this section covers several mind/body techniques that can be useful as part of a positive lifestyle.

Biofeedback

Several forms of biofeedback may be useful in promoting relaxation and stress reduction. Techniques include deep breathing, progressive muscle relaxation, or meditation.

A heart rate monitor may assist in some relaxation exercises. In one study conducted in my lab, taking a "10-Minute Timeout" which consisted of sitting quietly, clearing your mind, and focusing on lowering your heart rate on the monitor while gently thinking *down, down, down*, resulted in measurable stress relief. Heart monitors are also very useful in promoting heart health and safety when used to monitor aerobic physical activity using target heart rate zones. Such biofeedback is effective in enhancing a number of stress-reduction and exercise techniques.

Tai chi

This ancient Chinese discipline combines movement, deep breathing, and meditation, is appropriate for all ages, and can be adapted to all fitness levels. As your physical conditioning progresses, you can progress in the difficulty or duration of the tai chi exercises.

Studies show that tai chi may be particularly useful in helping older patients improve balance, strength, flexibility, and cardiovascular fitness. Recognizing its benefits, many medical health centers provide tai chi classes as part of their wellness programs.

Yoga

Yoga, which originated in India, combines movement (including stretching and poses) with breathing exercises and meditation to achieve relaxation and better flexibility, muscle strength, and functional health. Among the many styles of yoga are gentle forms that are appropriate for people with heart disease and perhaps other physical limitations. One benefit of yoga is that you can advance as your conditioning improves. Many medical health centers provide yoga classes as part of their wellness and rehabilitation programs.

Individuals with heart disease need to avoid beginning yoga with one of the newly popular forms that emphasize rigorous, aerobic workouts (often in a high heat and humid environment). Instead, start with a gentle, relaxation-oriented class tailored to beginners.

Therapeutic massage

Studies have shown that massage therapy performed by trained, certified massage therapists may help some individuals lower blood pressure and stress. Massage promotes relaxation, which in turn contributes to vasodilation (relaxation of the blood vessels) for some people.

If you are taking anti-clotting medicine, you probably want to avoid intense or deep massage, which might lead to bleeding or bruising; talk to your doctor first about suitability or cautions for you.

Opening up to spirituality

Although it may be splitting hairs, I separate spirituality from mind/body techniques. Both, however, are aspects of your psychological makeup. The degree of importance spirituality has on your outlook on life and perhaps even on your cardiovascular health is amazing. Two cases in point:

- ✔ **The power of prayer:** One recent study revealed that more than 95 percent of the people undergoing coronary artery bypass grafting engaged in prayer the evening before. I think placing more emphasis on understanding and respecting the spirituality of patients in modern cardiovascular medicine is not only good for healthcare givers as human beings but also enhances the outcomes of many of the procedures that they undertake.

- ✔ **The power of gardening:** Major studies show that people who garden regularly lower their risk of heart disease. Although gardeners may get a little exercise every day, it typically isn't enough to account for all the benefit. I think on some profound level, gardeners are getting a dose of spirituality as they tend other living things. Gardeners are optimists who plant seeds in spring, confident of the crops they'll produce in the summer and fall. Without a doubt, my patients who are gardeners seem to do better than the ones who don't have this connection with life and the earth.

Volunteering

My favorite song in the Disney movie *The Lion King* is "Circle of Life." This song reminds me that everyone is connected to each other in the circle of life. Recent studies show that people who work as volunteers and help others actually improve their own health. Isn't it wonderful to know that following your natural inclination to connect with other people and do good generates better health as a totally unintended side benefit?

Is natural better?

In recent years, natural products have developed quite a stamp of approval. Now, I'm all for natural products. Eating fruits and vegetables is the most natural way of getting fiber and many antioxidants and vitamins, particularly vitamin C.

Some of the most important drugs were developed from plant sources. You may even have growing in your garden now foxglove, the source of digitalis, one of the first and most important medicines for heart rhythm problem. The foxglove plants brightening your yard used to be ground up to produce a powder containing digitalis. Scientists later were able achieve even better results by purifying these same compounds in the laboratory. So the current medication known as *digoxin* leads straight back to foxglove and shares the same chemistry.

That leads to my last point: Just because a product is natural doesn't mean that it's better than a similar product that has been synthesized. Natural is neutral. Simply describing a product as "natural" does not qualify it as beneficial or ineffective nor as safe or harmful. Natural products, by their nature, haven't been subjected to the same purification processes that other products (approved medicines included) have undergone. That doesn't mean all natural products should be avoided. On the contrary, it simply means that consumers need to be aware that natural does not necessarily mean better or safer. Likewise, synthesized does not necessarily mean a product is not natural, that it doesn't have natural origins, or that it doesn't have side effects. As always, do your homework and use your common sense.

Looking at How Natural Supplements May Help or Harm

Ten years ago, I would've joined most physicians in saying that if you eat a balanced and healthy diet and meet all of the recommended daily allowances of vitamins and minerals, you probably don't need any supplements. However, within only the last five years, a number of studies have persuaded me that there are situations in which supplementation may be appropriate. At the same time, there are herbal products that may interact with other medications and cause potentially serious problems. As you can see, many issues still need to be explored.

So I recommend that you consider supplementation on a case-by-case basis and that you explore the issues with your cardiologist before taking any supplements. In addition, find out as much as you can about any given supplement and its potential role in cardiovascular and total health and its potential for negative interaction with other medicines you may be taking.

The sections that follow discuss some of the more popular natural supplements currently available and whether enough evidence exists to recommend them as substances that can lower your risk of heart disease or play a role in helping you fight heart disease.

Red yeast rice (monascus purpureus)

Red yeast rice contains an active agent known as *monascus purpureus* that comes from the ancient Chinese herbal medicine chest and recently was subjected to rigorous trials by Western science. The results are impressive. In fact, they're so impressive that the U.S. Food and Drug Administration (FDA) classified monascus purpureus as a drug that is pharmacologically related to the class of cholesterol-lowering drugs called *statins*. Because the FDA considers it a powerful drug, red yeast rice may no longer be sold legally in the United States as a food supplement. The best advice is to avoid taking this supplement. Because it is really a statin, you are almost certainly better off taking an FDA approved statin pill instead of the much less standardized red yeast rice.

Garlic

Beloved in all the world's cuisines, garlic was touted for its medicinal benefits more than 5,000 years ago in Sanskrit records from ancient India. Hippocrates wrote about garlic's use, and so did the Chinese. In recent years and currently, a number of studies tested or are testing the potential effect of garlic in many forms (raw, powdered, aged extract, and so on) on slowing atherosclerosis. Results to date are mixed. One of the difficulties is that the garlic preparations differ so greatly. Studies have also looked at the ability of garlic preparations to lower cholesterol, inhibit blood clotting, and blood pressure. Again, results are mixed.

For now, the jury is out on garlic as a beneficial cardiovascular supplement and research continues. If you're among the many people who enjoy the taste of garlic, cooking with it certainly can't hurt and may help, but I wouldn't recommend taking any garlic supplements in pill or powdered form without first discussing it with your cardiologist or primary-care physician.

Soluble fiber

Soluble fiber combines with water and fluids in the intestine to form gels that can absorb other substances and trap them. The trapped substances include bile acids that contain large amounts of cholesterol. Thus, consuming soluble fiber is a particularly good way of lowering cholesterol, because as bile acids are excreted from the body, the liver uses up cholesterol to make more bile acids.

So much strong evidence supports this function of soluble fiber that the FDA allows certain foods that are rich in soluble fiber to claim that, when they're used in conjunction with a low-fat diet, they may further lower your risk of heart disease. Oatmeal and whole-oat, ready-to-eat cereals are perhaps the most prominent among such foods that are eaten regularly.

The American Heart Association and National Cancer Institute recommend consuming 25 grams of fiber daily. Most people consume only about 12 grams. Thus, I strongly recommend that you try to increase the amount of fiber in your diet. High-fiber foods such as bran, beans, oatmeal, and many cereals are excellent sources of fiber, and so are many fruits and vegetables. Some fiber supplements, such as Metamucil and Citrucel, also may help.

Soy protein

Some cultures have prized soy protein for its health benefits since ancient times. Modern science confirms that the type of protein found in soybeans has a complete set of *amino acids,* which are the building blocks for the body's protein. Soy protein also seems to lower cholesterol and is thought to carry antioxidants that may help prevent heart disease in ways other than simply by lowering cholesterol levels. If you enjoy the taste of soy, you can consume extra soy protein by drinking soybean milk, using soy-based meat substitutes, or sampling the many new soy products that recently entered the marketplace. However, be aware that eating too much soy may produce a lot of intestinal gas and even diarrhea; so add soy products slowly to your diet.

Fish oil

Why do certain cultures that consume large quantities of cold-water fish (the Eskimo culture, for instance) have low incidences of heart disease? The reason seems related to the oils that these fish contain. These oils are high in a substance called omega-3 fatty acids. A number of studies show that cholesterol levels can be lowered by as much as 10 percent when fish is substituted for red meat in the diet two to three times per week. What a good reason to enjoy fish. I strongly recommend it. You'll get an excellent source of high-level protein that may, in addition, contain these cholesterol-lowering substances. One word of caution, however: Evidence is inconclusive about the benefits of taking fish oil supplements rather than actually eating the fish.

Antioxidant vitamin supplements

Antioxidants are thought to decrease the likelihood that LDL cholesterol will be oxidized. Research has focused particularly on vitamin C, vitamin E, and beta-carotene (vitamin A). But to date, the research has not found that these antioxidants in supplement form provide clinically significant benefits. For people with certain heart conditions, beta-carotene also appears to carry a risk.

The association of antioxidant vitamins with cardiac health observed in population studies may derive from the combined nutrients and micronutrients in whole foods. So what would I do? First, I encourage patients to eat a diet rich in fruits and vegetables because these are excellent sources of many nutrients, including antioxidants. To those who do not have contraindications (reasons they shouldn't use them) and would like to try supplements, I say that I don't object to their taking antioxidants, but I also point out that research to date does not support supplement use as a heart disease preventive.

Herbal supplements that interact with heart medicines

Research into certain herbal products has shown that they have pharmaco-active properties. That means that they act in the body like drugs. (Remember that many recognized prescription drugs have botanical roots or sources.) Therefore, some of these herbals can interact negatively with many medicines prescribed for various heart conditions. For that reasons, it is very important that, if you have risk factors for heart disease such as high blood pressure or diabetes or have coronary heart disease, heart failure, or other heart problems, you discuss all the issues with your primary-care doctor or cardiologist before taking any herbal products.

Among popular herbals, for example, ginkgo biloba, ginseng, hawthorn, and many others, may increase risk of bleeding if you take blood thinner medication such as warfarin because the herbals also have anticlotting properties. Another popular herbal, St. John's Wort, affects an enzyme that helps the body metabolize many cardiac drugs, so taking both may result in an overdose or underdose of your prescribed medicines. The bottom line for safety then: Always discuss herbal supplements with your physician before you take them.

Commonsense checklist for evaluating alternative therapies

So how do you sort through all the claims, evidence, information, and sometimes heated rhetoric about particular alternative products or techniques? Asking these questions may help you find and evaluate the information you need to make wise decisions:

🖝 When researching a specific therapy (particularly a controversial one), have you reviewed the arguments and evidence from all sides of the issue?

🖝 What evidence supports the effectiveness of the therapy?

Have scientific trials been conducted or is the support based only on testimony and anecdote?

Is the support based on quantifiable data or opinion?

How old, how large, and how well-designed were any scientific trials? (Good science always pushes the envelope, reevaluates, seeks to acquire more data, and, when necessary, changes its mind. A few scientific trials from the 1920s or 1950s that are unsupported by more recent studies or that are even contradicted by later studies would not be the best evidence of the effectiveness of a given substance or technique.)

🖝 How safe is the therapy?

Is there concrete evidence (not just a provider's or recipient's opinion) that the benefits outweigh the risks?

Does evidence suggest that the product does no harm when used as directed?

Under what conditions is service or treatment delivered?

🖝 What credentials and expertise does the practitioner of an alternative therapy or developer of a product have? (A mail-order PhD from a diploma mill won't inspire confidence in the developer of the "SuperDooper Mighty-Mineral Supplement," will it?)

🖝 What is the cost of the treatment or product?

🖝 Have you discussed the therapy with your primary-care physician and cardiologist? If you're actually using the therapy, have you told your doctor? Your doctor needs a complete picture to give you the best health-care, including guarding against negative interactions with your other medicines or therapies. Many doctors are also good sources of information.

Chapter 15

Taking Back Your Life after a Heart Event

A diagnosis of heart disease isn't the end of life as you know it; it just feels like it. A heart attack or heart surgery may feel like the end of the world, but your life and your health can emerge from these blows stronger than ever. That's where cardiac rehabilitation becomes important. If you or a family member has had a diagnosis of coronary heart disease (CHD) or a heart event, don't miss out on the following benefits of cardiac rehabilitation programs:

- Improved exercise tolerance and ability to carry out activities of daily living

- Reduced symptoms such as angina and shortness of breath

- Improved cholesterol and blood lipid levels

- Reduced cigarette smoking

- Improved sense of well-being

- Reduced stress

- Reduced mortality. Heart attack victims who participate in rehabilitation programs experience a 25 percent reduction in mortality during the first three years after their heart attacks when compared with those who don't participate.

Understanding Cardiac Rehabilitation

Cardiac rehabilitation is a long-term program with several therapeutic components designed to help individuals get better after a variety of heart problems, angioplasty, or cardiac surgery. It is an important tool in what physicians call *secondary prevention* of heart disease, which is prevention of another heart event after you've had one. The goal is nothing less than to help you get your life back.

Looking at the components of cardiac rehabilitation

Although tailored to the needs of each patient, all cardiac rehabilitation programs should include these four components, which I explain in detail later in the chapter:

- ✔ Education about your cardiac condition and treatment
- ✔ Exercise training and physical activity prescriptions
- ✔ Lifestyle modifications to reduce risk factors for heart disease
- ✔ Counseling and support

Although individual prescriptions for cardiac rehabilitation vary according to each individual patient's condition, the goals and benefits always remain the same:

- ✔ Educating you about how to control your cardiac condition
- ✔ Reducing the heart's disability and improving its ability to function in a way that supports your ability to carry out life's daily activities effectively and independently
- ✔ Decreasing the likelihood that you'll experience further problems from your cardiac condition and perhaps even decreasing the need for heart medicines
- ✔ Identifying and providing ways to modify risk factors that may result in continued problems from various forms of heart disease
- ✔ Increasing the likelihood that you will return to work and a full, happy, and long life following a cardiac event

Discovering just who needs cardiac rehabilitation

Modern cardiac rehabilitation programs are an important component of an overall care plan for many patients with heart disease and, more specifically, in these seven circumstances:

- ✔ When diagnosed with coronary heart disease/angina
- ✔ Following a heart attack
- ✔ Following coronary artery bypass surgery
- ✔ Following coronary angioplasty
- ✔ Following heart surgery on the valves
- ✔ Before and following heart transplantation
- ✔ When experiencing heart failure

As you can see from this list, the vast majority of people with heart disease can benefit from cardiac rehabilitation.

Exploring Varied Cardiac Rehabilitation Components

Formal, medically supervised cardiac rehabilitation programs usually take place either in the hospital or in the community. These programs offer a great advantage: Everything you need to improve your cardiac health can be found in one place, and knowledgeable medical staff members are on hand at all times to provide you with educational support, ensure your safety, and keep you motivated.

If you've been hospitalized for a heart attack, cardiac surgery, or other problem, your rehabilitation program typically starts while you're in the hospital. After you're discharged, you typically continue your program on an outpatient basis by participating in either a hospital- or community-sponsored cardiac rehabilitation program.

Unfortunately, some people are unable to participate in formal cardiac rehabilitation programs, because they live so far away from the centers where programs are provided. With advancing communications technology, many hospitals and cardiologists are beginning to offer home-based rehabilitation programs that use smart phone and online monitoring, supervision, and communication with participants. Such home-based programs are intended only for people who are at low or moderate risk of developing further problems.

Ideally, you will continue to work on your *rehab* for the rest of your life, because the information, strategies, and techniques you use during formal rehabilitation give you excellent tools for living long and well overall and not just for retooling the old ticker. That said, formal cardiac rehabilitation programs usually have three phases:

1. **Rehabilitation during hospitalization**
2. **Formal supervised rehabilitation program during recovery**
3. **Maintenance program**

Starting rehabilitation while you're in the hospital

If you're hospitalized for a cardiac problem or surgery, your rehabilitation begins during your stay in the hospital.

Members of the rehabilitation team begin counseling you on your cardiac condition and how to manage it. Topics may include nutrition, weight reduction (if necessary), stress reduction, stopping smoking, and other lifestyle modifications. You also begin supervised physical therapy and physical activity.

When doctors decide you are ready to go home, your medical team makes sure that you receive instructions for what you need to do at home to continue your progress. Your doctor usually recommends when you should begin a medically supervised cardiac rehabilitation program. The timing depends on your particular situation and condition, but, in general, you'll be ready to start in one to six weeks.

In the meantime, you're not supposed to be idle at home. You need to continue with the physical activities, exercises, and diet your physician recommends for your recovery. In some instances, your physician may prescribe home visits from a social worker or physical therapist to help you out. Health insurance will often pay for such visits for a short period after hospitalization; check your policy.

Continuing rehabilitation during recovery

After your initial recovery, you begin participating in a medically supervised cardiac rehabilitation program. Typical cardiac rehabilitation programs feature group and individual exercises, along with a variety of educational programs that help lower your risk factors for heart disease.

Your physical activity usually includes aerobic exercise on a treadmill, a stationary cycle, or a walking track. However, equipment and activities also are available for people with walking difficulties to build their aerobic capacity. Enhancing mobility is, after all, a goal. The physical activity starts slowly to ensure safety but gradually builds to a more intensive program.

During your exercise program, your heart rate, blood pressure, and, at least in the early stages, electrical impulses and rhythm of your heart as indicated by an electrocardiogram (ECG) are monitored by a nurse or other healthcare professional to make sure you're not having any problems.

Strength training, in some instances, may be included in your program. Proper instruction and supervision are crucial, and strength training is not advised for all cardiac conditions.

Most rehabilitation programs include classes in nutrition, risk-factor reduction, weight management (if necessary), smoking cessation, and stress management education. Access to counseling, educational materials, and support groups also is likely to be available for

- ✔ Job and vocational guidance to help you with returning to work

- ✔ Physical capabilities and limitations, including (but not limited to) when you can start having sexual relations, how much exertion you can take in daily life, and so on

- ✔ Psychological and emotional matters

Although your physician recommends the length of time you should participate in a cardiac rehabilitation program, 6 to 12 weeks usually is the minimum. A number of studies, however, indicate that heart rehab patients who participate for periods of from three to six months to a year experience even greater improvements.

Another benefit of cardiac rehab is that you and your family receive support and encouragement from the cardiac rehab team and other participants in the program. This support lets you know that you and your family are not alone and helps ease the anxiety and depression that are normal after a heart event or diagnosis of a problem.

Maintaining your program to keep gaining benefits

Continuing your physical activity program and sustaining and strengthening your new nutritional and lifestyle practices are important for maintaining and increasing the gains you achieve during your formal rehab program. In fact, "keeping on keeping on" is the key to unlocking the lasting benefits of cardiac rehabilitation. Some medical centers have maintenance classes that you may continue to attend, or you may find a program at a community center.

Educating Yourself about Your Heart Condition

Being diagnosed with heart disease, experiencing a heart attack, or undergoing heart surgery is scary. In fact, it's so scary that you may try to avoid thinking about your condition — you just want to get over it and get back to your old life. Or it's so scary that thinking positively about the future is difficult. Fear, denial, anger, and all the other emotional reactions to heart disease or a cardiac event are normal. The first and foremost tool for dealing with them is knowledge. That's why helping you educate yourself about your particular condition is an important component of rehabilitation programs.

Finding out as much as you can about your condition, how to manage it, how to reduce any resulting limitations, and how to enhance abilities can unlock the door to a new freedom and a new discovery of what having a good life truly means. If you've had a heart event, the information in this book (in conjunction with the rehabilitation prescribed by your doctor) can help you become a knowledgeable, educated patient who is empowered to become an equal partner in his or her recovery and rehabilitation.

Exercise and Physical Activity as Part of Rehabilitation

Slowly progressive exercise training and physical activity programs and prescriptions represent the cornerstone of all modern cardiac rehabilitation programs. The benefits of such activity for people with heart disease are numerous, including

✔ Increasing the efficiency and performance of the heart muscle itself.

✔ Increasing the efficiency of the exercising muscles, thereby reducing the heart's workload.

✔ Reducing the likelihood of further cardiac problems. This benefit is particularly true when such exercise programs are combined with risk-factor reduction and psychological support.

✔ Increasing your exercise capacity, which in turn can significantly improve your quality of life and result in a variety of other psychological benefits.

✔ Helping you feel that you're playing an active role in your recovery from heart disease.

Remember that, as functional capacity increases after an acute heart problem, the likelihood of your returning to work and favorite activities increases.

Progressive exercise programs may also combat other risk factors for heart disease. For example, regular physical activity can significantly increase high-density lipoprotein (HDL — the good cholesterol), which is associated with decreased cardiac problems. In addition, regular physical activity can help with weight loss and may lower low-density lipoprotein (LDL — the bad kind of cholesterol), thereby further lowering the risk of future cardiac problems. (For more about cholesterol, check out Chapter 9.)

Getting started on an exercise program for rehab

In many instances, your doctor may require that you undergo some form of exercise tolerance test as part of the early process of cardiac rehabilitation. During that test, your doctor looks for evidence of inadequate blood flow to the heart, abnormal heart rhythms, or inadequate pumping action by the heart during exercise. Armed with this information, the doctor and other healthcare workers can develop an individualized exercise program that enables you to achieve maximum benefits from exercise, while ensuring maximum safety.

After you suffer a cardiac event, exercise factors such as duration, intensity, and frequency of exercise are monitored carefully to ensure your safety as you begin exercising. Monitoring these factors ensures that your exercise program follows a slow progression toward helping to maximize your functional capacity and encouraging you to adopt a safe program that can be carried on for the rest of your life.

Modifying rehabilitative exercise training for specific conditions

Although basic principles of exercise training apply to all cardiac rehabilitation, some people with specific conditions require various modifications to the basic exercise-training program.

Patients with heart failure

Exercise programs in cardiac rehabilitation can be extremely helpful for people experiencing heart failure. Some studies show that people suffering from heart failure can improve their exercise capacity between 25 percent and 30 percent through controlled exercise programs. With those improvements typically come other improvements in the form of a better quality of life and decreased symptoms. The exercise prescription, however, needs to be modified in patients with heart failure because of their limited endurance. Lower target heart rates and intermittent rest periods enable them to slowly increase their endurance. Heart rates during exercise sessions typically are set at 10 beats per minute below the level at which any evidence of shortness of breath occurs.

The elderly

People older than 65 who have cardiac problems and participate in cardiac rehabilitation can achieve significant improvements in their capacity to conduct activities of daily living. In one study, functional capacity increased by 50 percent. Although exercise programs may need to be modified to accommodate limited endurance, elderly individuals stand to gain the most from cardiac rehabilitation. Yet this group nevertheless is among the most underserved.

Patients with heart rhythm problems

Patients who have been hospitalized with heart rhythm problems may benefit from cardiac rehabilitation programs. Because these people may be at particularly high risk for problems during cardiac rehabilitation, however, they require

✔ Supervision by doctors who are knowledgeable about their specific rhythm problems

✔ Appropriate medications to suppress rhythm disturbances

✔ Longer periods of continuous monitoring (using electrocardiograms) than individuals who haven't had cardiac rhythm problems

Women

Although women experience the same benefits of exercise training as men do during cardiac rehabilitation, women are significantly less likely to be referred for cardiac rehabilitation and when referred they are less likely to attend. This shortfall is particularly unfortunate because about half of all deaths from coronary heart disease now occur in women. Women are also more likely than men to experience other problems, including death, following a heart attack. Thus, cardiac rehabilitation is particularly important for women. So, ladies, insist on it or find out why it isn't recommended.

Cardiac transplantation patients

Research shows that cardiac rehabilitation is highly effective for cardiac transplantation patients, helping increase their endurance and capacity to perform activities of daily living.

A number of changes in the cardiovascular system occur following cardiac transplantation. These changes often require modifications to typical cardiac rehabilitation programs. For example, the response of a transplanted heart to exercise is different in terms of heart rate than in a nontransplanted heart. During the transplantation process, all the nerves that serve the normal heart are severed. The result is a difference in how the reattached nerves send signals to the heart. Therefore, heart transplant patients need to be involved in programs with an experienced rehabilitation team whose members are skilled in their particular exercise prescription.

Developing Strategies for Long-Term Success

How successful any rehabilitation program is in lowering your risk of future cardiac events relates directly to how conscientiously you follow the program.

Cardiac rehabilitation has many benefits and minimal risks. Comprehensive cardiac rehabilitation programs help you or a loved one fight back against heart disease. The biggest risk is not participating at all. Ask your doctor whether cardiac rehabilitation is appropriate for you, and when it is, take advantage of this potentially lifesaving part of modern cardiac care.

Assessing in your own mind and heart, discussing all the potential benefits of cardiac rehabilitation with your family and physician, and developing a strategy for sticking with it in the long run (or long walk!) are important steps to take. The formal rehabilitation program may end, but your work is never done.

Modifying your lifestyle to reduce the risks of additional heart problems

Risk-factor reduction is particularly important for patients who have heart disease, have had a heart attack, and/or have undergone cardiac surgery. Cardiac rehabilitation programs place particular emphasis on blood pressure control, proper nutritional counseling, weight reduction (if the patient is overweight), and smoking cessation. Here are the details:

- ✔ **Blood pressure control:** Managing your blood pressure by keeping it within normal levels can reduce your risk of further problems and complications from your heart disease. Adhering to a multifaceted approach that includes education, diet modifications, a program of physical activity, stress reduction, and prescribed medications is important. (For more about hypertension, see Chapter 8.)

- ✔ **Nutritional counseling:** Strong evidence exists that lowering blood cholesterol and improving lipoprotein profiles are extremely beneficial for people with heart disease and those who have had a heart attack, angioplasty, or any surgery, including bypass grafting. Seeking such nutritional instruction from a registered dietitian can be very helpful. Remember, sodium-restricted diets are appropriate for patients with high blood pressure or heart failure.

- ✔ **Weight control:** Studies show that losing weight and maintaining weight at appropriate levels can help people with heart disease control high blood pressure, improve and even normalize their cholesterol levels, and control the risk of diabetes. Weight loss also contributes to improving your ability to comfortably carry out daily activities (see Chapter 10).

- ✔ **Smoking cessation:** Without a doubt, patients with heart disease who continue to smoke have a higher likelihood of suffering further complications or even death. The converse also is also true. Patients who stop smoking after a heart attack reduce their risk of further cardiac events. (See Chapter 11 for information and strategies on quitting smoking.)

Getting some counseling and support

The majority of patients who've suffered an acute problem from heart disease experience one or more psychological problems. Common conditions include

✔ **Moderate to severe depression:** Following a heart attack, up to 20 percent of patients experience this kind of depression. Likewise, up to 10 percent of them face significant anxiety disorders that require therapy.

✔ **A reduction in sexual activity:** In fact, almost 25 percent of heart attack patients never resume sexual activity and more than 50 percent decrease their sexual activity following a heart attack.

✔ **Family and marital problems and social isolation:** These problems are common sequels to heart disease.

People with severe heart disease commonly go through a cycle of fear that often leads to anger and ultimately to depression. Some of the more common feelings are

✔ Fear that you're dying

✔ Fear that chest pains will recur

✔ Fear that you'll never return to work

✔ Fear that you'll never have sex again

✔ Anger that a heart problem happened to you

✔ Anger at yourself for not changing conditions that may or may not have been under your control that ultimately resulted in the heart problem

✔ Anger with family and friends

✔ Depression at the thought that your "life is over" (or will never be the same again)

✔ Depression at the idea that others may think you're weak or damaged goods

Psychological counseling can help in all of these situations, particularly during the early phases of recovery, and it therefore needs to be a part of all cardiac rehabilitation programs. Participating in a support group with other people who've experienced problems or have conditions similar to yours can be beneficial. Ask your cardiologist or a member of the staff at your rehabilitation center about groups in your area. You can also find support groups online.

Support from counselors also can help you establish positive interactive links with your family and friends. A number of rehab programs offer support groups and educational classes for family members that can enhance the recovery of your entire family. Yes, heart problems affect more than the victim who suffers from them.

Safely returning to work

One benefit of cardiac rehabilitation is that trained professionals can help guide anyone who has suffered from a heart problem in making important decisions, such as determining whether and when to return to work, choosing whether to change the type of work you do, and assessing the risks of having further problems if you return to work.

Your physician often is guided by the results of objective tests, such as the treadmill exercise test. The results of such tests, in conjunction with the physical demands of your job, help guide you and your medical team in deciding whether and when you return to work. The exact nature of your work, whether it involves strenuous labor, and particularly whether it involves work with your arms and chest, are important issues to discuss with your physician. Be sure that you talk to your doctor about the nature and levels of stress that are typical of your work.

The good news: Most people can return to work following most acute heart problems, and cardiac rehab helps that happen sooner.

Partnering with your physician

If you think you or a loved one is eligible for and can benefit from cardiac rehabilitation, *talk to your doctor.* If your doctor isn't willing to consider cardiac rehabilitation for you and you think you're eligible, obtaining a second opinion may be worthwhile.

Some questions to ask your doctor include

- Am I eligible for cardiac rehabilitation?
- Is cardiac rehabilitation covered by my health insurance?
- Where is the nearest cardiac rehabilitation program?
- How often do I need to go to cardiac rehabilitation sessions?
- How long should I participate in a cardiac rehabilitation program?
- What benefits can I expect from a cardiac rehabilitation program?

Part V
Heart-Healthy Recipes

5 Versatile, Heart-Healthy Seasonings

- **Lemon juice:** Lemon is a good source of vitamin C, potassium, and folate, and lemon juice (and lime juice) can enhance the flavor of many foods. Partner it with olive oil for salad dressing, or to season or make a sauce for fish, chicken, and pasta dishes. Squeeze it over fresh vegetables instead of butter and over fresh fruit to add zing and prevent discoloration.

- **Nuts:** Nuts can add great flavor and crunch to a variety of foods, and they're good sources of protein, omega-3 fats, dietary fiber, and vitamin E. Add chopped nuts to fruit and vegetable salads. Blend nuts into sauces (such as pesto) for fish, lean meats, and pasta. Use nut meal as part of coatings for baked chicken, pork, or fish. Add them to smoothies.

- **Garlic:** One of the world's oldest seasonings, garlic is also one of the most versatile. It's a good source of vitamin C, vitamin B6, manganese, calcium, phosphorus, and selenium. Use garlic in fresh or dried form.

- **Pepper:** This broad category includes black pepper and a variety of dried red chili peppers, like cayenne, chipotle, and ancho. Yes, black pepper is a seed, and chili peppers are vegetables, but both types bring spiciness and a range of heats to dishes ranging from simple dishes like scrambled eggs to complex dishes from most of the world's cuisines. Experiment with various peppers in low-fat dishes.

- **Natural-brewed soy sauce (low sodium):** Use real brewed soy sauce (shoyu, made from soy and wheat) in small amounts to add flavor to meat, vegetable, and grain dishes. It provides small amounts of several vitamins and minerals but is also high in sodium. It's biggest contribution is flavor. A tablespoon of soy in a pound of ground, 99 percent fat-free turkey breast, for instance, adds depth of flavor. If you can't eat wheat, tamari is typically made with soy alone.

web extras

Are your kitchen and pantry equipped for heart-healthy cooking? Check out the basic essentials at www.dummies.com/extras/preventingreversingheart disease.

In this part . . .

- ✔ Adopt a nutrient-rich, heart-healthy way of eating as a primary strategy for achieving healthy cholesterol levels, reaching optimal blood pressure levels, and maintaining a healthy weight.

- ✔ Swap high-fat, overly processed foods for whole grains, healthy fats, and lean proteins — without sacrificing taste.

- ✔ Find a variety of heart-healthy recipes for breakfast, lunch, dinner, snacks, and desserts.

Chapter 16

Heart-Healthy Breakfasts

● ●

In This Chapter

▶ Making breakfast dishes ahead of time to get you through several mornings

▶ Whipping up healthy 5-minute breakfasts

▶ Discovering heart-healthy recipes for leisurely breakfasts or brunches

● ●

Eating a good breakfast starts the day off right! A nutrient-rich breakfast gives your body the calories it needs to get going after the night's fast and meet the demands of an active day. Eating breakfast can also help you be more productive at school or at work. Numerous studies show that children and adults who eat breakfast typically have better cognitive performance in the morning than people who skip breakfast. For some people, but not all, skipping breakfast may contribute to weight gain. Why? Often, if you skip breakfast, you start feeling hungry mid-morning. Then it's easy to succumb to the temptation to fill up with a sweet or salty snack.

Breakfast is a great time for consuming fiber and fruits, too. Many people get up to 25 percent of their daily fiber at breakfast. The availability of high-fiber ready-to-eat cereals (that are lower in sugar and sodium, too) make increasing fiber consumption easier than ever. Better yet, eating fiber lowers your risk of heart disease. Eat a bowl of fruit or a slice of melon, cut a banana or add berries to your cereal, and drink a glass of fruit juice and you've made a great start to getting lots of fruit in your day.

The recipes in this chapter include quick breakfasts you can make in a few minutes, recipes you can make quickly in an evening and have ready to go for several mornings, and more extensive recipes for leisurely breakfasts on your days off. All will add taste and variety to your mornings and help you get a great start. The recipes come from my *Healthy Heart Cookbook For Dummies*, by yours truly, and *Mediterranean Diet Cookbook For Dummies*, by Meri Raffetto and Wendy Jo Peterson — two great resources for heart-healthy cooking.

Quick Breakfasts You Can Prepare in Advance

Is there a time crunch in the morning at your home? Well, duh! Of course there is. Our family has four children scrambling with their parents to get fueled up before dashing off to school and work. So I know about hectic mornings. The recipes in this section can add to your options for healthy breakfast foods that you can prepare ahead.

These recipes are easy to prepare ahead on the weekend or on a weekday night. Store the cooled muffins and scones in airtight containers and reheat them in a toaster oven (5 to 7 minutes) or in a microwave (10 seconds). Eat the granola like any ready-to-eat cereal with milk or yogurt, or store it in individual serving containers and eat it like trail mix.

For a complete breakfast that features several food groups, pair the muffins, scones, or granola with either the Fruit and Yogurt Smoothie or the Chocolate Banana Soy Shake (you can find the recipes in the later section "5-Minute Breakfasts for Those on the Go").

Mark's Low-Fat Oat Bran Muffins with Fresh Peaches

Prep time: 15 min • **Cook time:** 15 min • **Yield:** 12 muffins

Ingredients	Directions
2 cups oat bran	*1* Preheat oven to 425 degrees.
2 teaspoons baking powder	
1 teaspoon cinnamon	*2* Grease one 12-cup or two 6-cup muffin pan(s).
½ teaspoon kosher salt	*3* Combine the oat bran, baking powder, cinnamon, and salt in a mixing bowl and stir to blend.
1 cup milk	
2 egg whites	*4* In a separate mixing bowl, combine the milk, egg whites, canola oil, maple syrup, and peaches (or other fruit).
2 tablespoons canola oil	
½ cup maple syrup	
1 cup diced fresh peaches (or blueberries or diced strawberries)	*5* Pour the peach mixture into the dry ingredients and stir very gently, just to combine. Lumps in the batter are okay.
	6 Spoon batter into the muffin pan(s), filling about three-quarters full.
	7 Bake 15 minutes or until golden brown on top.

Per serving: Calories 117 (From fat 27); Total fat 3 g (Saturated 0 g); Protein 4 g; Carbohydrate 24 g (Dietary fiber 3 g); Cholesterol 0 mg; Sodium 184 mg.

Source: Healthy Heart Cookbook For Dummies

Peach Scones

Prep time: 30 min • **Cook time:** 12 min • **Yield:** 8 scones

Ingredients	Directions
2 cups flour	*1* Preheat oven to 425 degrees.
2 tablespoons sugar	
1 tablespoon baking power	*2* In a medium bowl, mix together flour, sugar, baking powder, baking soda, and salt.
1 teaspoon salt	
3 tablespoons butter	*3* Add the butter and cut it into the flour mixture using two forks. Mix until the butter is well-incorporated and the mixture gets crumbly. Add the peaches and almond extract, and stir to combine.
1 cup chopped peaches, fresh or canned, well drained	
½ teaspoon almond extract	
2 eggs	*4* In a small bowl, beat the eggs; whisk in the buttermilk. Pour the egg and milk mixture into the dry ingredients. Gently combine until moistened, gathering dough together into a ball. Set mixture aside for about 5 minutes.
½ cup fat-free buttermilk (or skim milk)	
1 tablespoon decorating or coarse sugar (optional)	
	5 Divide dough in half. On a floured surface shape each half into a circle, approximately ½-inch thick. Use your hands to gently pat out the dough. Cut each round of dough into four wedges.
	6 Place the wedges on a nonstick baking sheet. If desired, sprinkle with decorating or coarse sugar. Bake for about 12 minutes, or until lightly golden brown. Serve warm. Scones can be reheated in a toaster over.

Per serving: *Calories 206 (From fat 54); 6 g (Saturated 1 g); Protein 6 g; Carbohydrate 32 g (Dietary fiber 1 g); Cholesterol 54 mg; Sodium 557 mg.*

Tip: Keep scones in an air tight plastic bag or container. Eat within 2 or 3 days.

Source: Healthy Heart Cookbook For Dummies

Homemade Granola

Prep time: 15 min • **Cook time:** 45 min • **Yield:** Eight ½ cup servings

Ingredients	Directions
6⅓ cups rolled oats (regular, not instant)	**1** Preheat oven to 300 degrees.
2 tablespoons whole wheat flour	**2** In a large mixing bowl, combine the oats, flour, dry milks, sesame and sunflower seeds, almonds, lemon or orange zest, and ground cinnamon. Mix well.
3 tablespoons nonfat dry milk	
6 tablespoons sesame seeds	**3** In a small bowl, stir together the concentrated apply juice, hot water, and honey. Add the granola mixture, stirring occasionally.
6 tablespoons sunflower seeds	
6 tablespoons chopped almonds	**4** Thinly spread the mixture in a shallow baking pan. Bake until dry and toasted, about 40 to 45 minutes, stirring occasionally.
1 tablespoon lemon or orange zest, grated	
1 tablespoon ground cinnamon	**5** Pour into large mixing bowl and cool slightly before stirring in chopped dates and the currants.
½ cup unsweetened apple juice, frozen concentrate, thawed	**6** Cool completely before storing in tightly sealed plastic bags or glass jars. Store in a cool place. Use within 10 days.
½ cup hot water	
8 teaspoons honey	
½ cup chopped dates or granulated date sugar	
¾ cup currants, dried	

Per serving: Calories 311 (From fat 81); 9 g (Saturated 1 g); Protein 9 g; Carbohydrate 53 g (Dietary fiber 7 g); Cholesterol 0 mg; Sodium 20 mg.

Tip: For variety, mix ½ cup of granola with ½ cup of nonfat plain Greek yogurt. Add fresh berries or diced fresh fruit such as peaches or apples if you like.

Source: Healthy Heart Cookbook For Dummies

5-Minute Breakfasts for Those on the Go

Nutrient-rich smoothies and breakfast shakes can make up most of a good breakfast or lunch. Here are other ingredients that taste great in smoothies and add protein and/or healthful fats for a satisfying breakfast or lunch. If you like a lot of fresh fruit in your smoothies, these ingredients act as thickeners also:

- **Nonfat yogurt and cottage cheese:** These dairy foods are good sources of protein, calcium, and vitamin D

- **Silken tofu:** This soy food offers a good nondairy source of protein.

- **Nut butters and nuts:** Peanut butter, almonds and almond butter, walnuts, and other nuts offer good sources of protein and healthful oils.

- **Sesame seeds or tahini and other seeds:** These are good, non-tree-nut sources of proteins, healthful oils, and antioxidants. Other good seeds to try include pumpkin seeds, flax seed, and chia seeds.

Don't have time to whip up even a quick breakfast smoothie? Then try one of these super-quick but healthy breakfasts. Note that each includes at least three food groups to ensure a variety of heart-healthy nutrients:

- A whole-grain ready-to-eat cereal topped with fresh fruit, a few chopped nuts, and nonfat milk or nondairy milk

- A toasted whole-grain bagel or English muffin topped with 2 tablespoons of natural peanut butter and raisins, and to drink, a glass of nonfat milk or nondairy milk.

- A toasted whole-grain waffle "buttered" with 2 tablespoons of natural peanut butter and folded around a half of a banana; and to drink, a glass of nonfat milk or nondairy milk.

- Nonfat Greek yogurt topped with our Homemade Granola (see the recipe earlier in this chapter) or another low-fat granola, and fruit.

- A slice or two of cold cheese-and-veggie pizza and a glass of orange juice.

Fruit and Yogurt Smoothie

Prep time: 5 min • **Yield:** 2 smoothies

Ingredients	Directions
1 banana	**1** Combine all ingredients in a blender and blend until smooth and frothy.
½ frozen strawberries or peaches	
1 cup plain, nonfat yogurt	
¼ cup orange juice	

Per serving: Calories 152 (From fat 9); 1 g (Saturated 0 g); Protein 8g; Carbohydrate 30 g (Dietary fiber 3 g); Cholesterol 2 mg; Sodium 95 mg.

Tip: For a breakfast on the go, treat this recipe as one serving. Add a tablespoon of oat bran or wheat bran if you like.

Source: Healthy Heart Cookbook For Dummies

Kitchen essentials for preparing quick breakfasts

Having the right foods and right equipment on hand can ensure that you and your family members can quickly prepare a heart-healthy breakfast even if you have only 10 minutes.

In the pantry and refrigerator:

- ✔ Ready-to-eat whole grain cold cereals
- ✔ Quick cook (not instant) oatmeal and other hot cereals
- ✔ Frozen whole grain waffles
- ✔ Whole grain bread, bagels and/or English muffins
- ✔ Fresh fruit, such as bananas, apples, pears, and berries
- ✔ Fruit and vegetable juice — orange, grapefruit, tomato, mixed vegetable
- ✔ Nonfat milk or nondairy milk

Equipment:

- ✔ Toaster — four slot, suitable for toast, bagels and muffins
- ✔ Toaster oven
- ✔ Blender (if you have a big family and love smoothies, consider two)
- ✔ Microwave

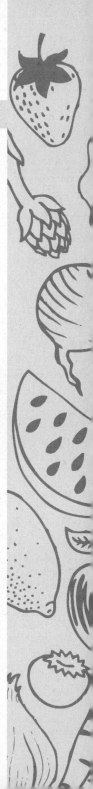

Chocolate Banana Soy Shake

Prep time: 5 min • **Yield:** 1 shake

Ingredients	*Directions*
1 large banana, cut into chunks	*1* Place banana chunks in freezer overnight or until completely frozen.
1 cup vanilla soy milk	
1 tablespoon chocolate syrup	*2* Combine all ingredients in a blender and blend until a smooth consistency is reached.
1 teaspoon smooth peanut butter	*3* Pour into a large glass and enjoy.

Per serving: Calories 279 (From fat 72); Total fat 8 g (Saturated 1 g); Protein 10 g; Carbohydrate 48 g (Dietary fiber 7 g); Cholesterol 0 mg; Sodium 74 mg.

Tip: After you have made this shake two or three times by the recipe, try experimenting with your own combinations of fruit and soy milk.

Source: Healthy Heart Cookbook For Dummies

Go for coffee and tea

Does your day start with a hot cup of coffee or tea? Do your eyes droop with sleep until that first lovely sip goes down your throat? Does it take a second cup to really rev your motor? Do you wonder if this regular consumption of coffee or tea is good or bad for you?

Wonder no more. The most recent studies indicate that both coffee and tea appear to contribute to health when consumed in ways that don't add a lot of extra calories. Both coffee and tea (green, black, oolong) are loaded with antioxidants and flavanoids that support heart health and total health.

Studies in coffee found no problem with drinking up to six 8-ounce cups daily. Just remember that the most popular size in most java joints is the 16-ounce large or grande. Benefits studied were in black coffee. Adding sugar, cream, and flavored syrups can add hundreds of empty calories.

Regular tea *(Camellia sinensis),* as found in green, black, white, and oolong varieties, also abounds with healthful antioxidants, such as catechins. Tea is also lower in caffeine than coffee. Drinking your favorite type hot or cold can contribute to a healthy diet. Just avoid adding caloric sweeteners and flavorings; that tip would exclude most bottled varieties.

What about herbal teas? There are many different varieties and scientific study has not been extensive yet. A number of popular herbal teas such as hibiscus, chamomile, and rooibos (red bush tea) appear to be safe. But hundreds of different herbs used in teas have not been studied. Always consult your healthcare provider before drinking any "medicinal" herbal teas.

Greek Yogurt and Fruit Bowls

Prep time: 10 min • **Yield:** 4 servings

Ingredients	Directions
2 cups red or green grapes **4 fresh apricots**	*1* Slice the grapes in half and divide into 4 bowls (½ cup per bowl). Slice the apricots and discard the seeds; divide equally into the 4 bowls.
2 cups low-fat plain Greek yogurt **4 tablespoons slivered almonds**	*2* Top each fruit bowl with ½ cup low-fat Greek yogurt and sprinkle with the slivered almonds and oats.
4 tablespoons raw, old fashioned oats **4 tablespoons honey**	*3* Drizzle 1 tablespoon of honey over each bowl and serve.

Per serving: Calories 206 (From Fat 45); Total fat 5 g (Saturated 0 g); Protein 8 g; Carbohydrate 36 g (Dietary fiber 3 g); Cholesterol 0 mg; Sodium 23 mg.

Source: Mediterranean Diet Cookbook For Dummies

Going Greek for Yogurt

Greek yogurt has skyrocketed in popularity. While both Greek nonfat yogurt and regular nonfat yogurt offer great taste and nutrition, there are several reasons you may wish to choose a Greek yogurt. Just remember to choose nonfat or low-fat because regular is high in saturated fat.

Creamier texture. Most people find that Greek yogurts have a creamier, thicker texture than regular yogurt. Try different brands to find the one you like best.

Higher protein. Because Greek yogurt is strained to remove liquid whey and make it thicker, the amount of protein increases to about 15-20 grams in a 6-ounce serving compared to about 9 grams in the same size serving of regular yogurt.

Lower sugar content. Straining also lowers the amount of lactose (milk sugar) in Greek yogurt compared to regular yogurt. Beware, however, of Greek yogurt (or regular yogurt) that's been sweetened with fruit jams or other added sweeteners.

Leisurely Breakfasts and Brunches

On your days off and on vacation days, you have time to enjoy a more leisurely breakfast. These are also great times to entertain friends and family for brunch. The recipes in this section take a little more time to prepare. The payoff comes when you enjoy their wonderful taste while knowing just how good they are for you.

These recipes, you'll also notice, include eggs. The most recent research suggests that eating up to one egg daily does not contribute to elevated cholesterol for most people. If you have diabetes or heart disease, your doctor may recommend that you limit your whole egg intake to three or four per week. Why not experiment with using egg substitute in the recipes that use beaten eggs?

These recipes also contain more fat than the many of the other recipes in this chapter. However, you'll notice that very little is saturated fat, and a good bit comes from healthful olive oil. Eaten occasionally, these recipes certainly fit within a heart-healthy diet.

For an enjoyable way of healthy eating that you can adopt for a lifetime, I think you have to take this old saying to heart: *moderation in all things, including moderation.* This proverb is often attributed to a first-century Roman named Petronius. One thing you can say about the Romans is that they knew how to throw a banquet. So as you are thinking about a heart-healthy approach to eating, make room for some "feasts," including brunches that feature recipes like the ones I include in this section.

Mediterranean Egg Scramble

Prep time: 15 min • **Cook time:** 25 min • **Yield:** 4 servings

Ingredients	Directions
1 teaspoon olive oil	*1* In a large nonstick skillet, heat the olive oil and butter to medium-high heat. Add the sliced potatoes and sauté for about 15 minutes or until golden. Add the bell pepper and olives and cook for 4 minutes.
1 teaspoon butter	
3 medium-sized new potatoes, thinly sliced	
¼ large red bell pepper, small diced	*2* In a medium bowl, whisk together the parsley, ricotta, and eggs. Pour the egg mixture over the potato mixture, stirring every 30 seconds until firm and set but not dry, about 3 minutes. Salt and pepper the egg scramble to taste.
8 black olives, chopped	
¼ cup fresh parsley, chopped	
¼ cup fresh ricotta cheese	*3* Serve with crusty bread, lightly toasted and buttered with 1 teaspoon of butter or lightly brushed with 1 teaspoon of extra-virgin olive oil per slice.
6 eggs	
Salt and pepper to taste	
4 slices crusty bread	
4 teaspoons butter or extra virgin olive oil	

Per Serving: Calories 330 (From fat 113); Total fat 13 g (Saturated 3 g); Protein 13 g; Carbohydrate 43 g (Dietary fiber 4 g); Cholesterol 9 mg; Sodium 364 mg.

Vary It! Replace these vegetables with artichoke hearts and fennel for an Italian scramble.

Tip: Though not in the original recipe, you can make this recipe even more heart healthy by selecting a sourdough or wholegrain bread for the toast.

Source: Mediterranean Diet Cookbook For Dummies

Eggs Benedict with Asparagus and Low-Fat Hollandaise Sauce

Prep time: 20 min • **Cook time:** 15 min • **Yield:** 4 servings

Ingredients	*Directions*
4 English muffins	**1** Split English muffins and toast.
8 large eggs	
8½-ounce Canadian bacon slices	**2** Place asparagus spears in a steamer and steam for 3 to 5 minutes, depending on their thickness. They should be tender but firm.
½ cup Low-Fat Hollandaise Sauce (see the recipe that follows)	**3** While the muffins are toasting and the asparagus is steaming, crack each egg individually and carefully into a large nonstick skillet filled with ½ inch simmering water. Cover and cook for 2 to 3 minutes or until the egg whites are firm and opaque white.
16 asparagus spears	
Salt and pepper to taste	
4 cups freshly squeezed orange juice	**4** Warm the Canadian bacon slices in a medium sauté pan over medium heat, about 1 minute per side. Place 2 English muffin halves on each plate and top each half with a slice of bacon.
	5 When the eggs are ready, drain and place over the bacon. Place 4 asparagus spears between the muffins on each plate. Season the top of the eggs and the asparagus with salt and pepper. Top each muffin with 1 tablespoon Low-Fat Hollandaise Sauce. Serve immediately with 1 cup freshly squeezed orange juice per person.

Low-Fat Hollandaise Sauce

¼ **cup homemade or canned chicken broth or stock**

¼ **cup fresh lemon juice**

½ **cup liquid egg substitute**

2 teaspoons canola oil

¼ **teaspoon mustard**

Salt and pepper to taste

1 In a medium saucepan, bring the broth and lemon juice to a rolling boil. Allow to boil about 4 to 6 minutes or until liquid volume is reduced by half.

2 While the broth and lemon juice are reducing, whisk the egg substitute in a medium stainless steel or glass bowl until the egg triples in volume. You can use a hand-mixer or a standing mixer to do this.

3 When the broth has reduced, whisk in the oil and the mustard. Then *slowly* add the reduced broth to the egg mixture, whisking the entire time. Season with salt and pepper to taste.

4 The sauce will thicken as it sits and cools; make it immediately before serving, or if you make it ahead of time, warm it over low heat while whisking to thin the sauce.

Per serving: Calories 491 (From fat 144); Total fat 16 g (Saturated 4 g); Protein 29 g; Carbohydrate 55 g (Dietary fiber 3 g); Cholesterol 436 mg; Sodium 994 mg.

Tip: If you don't have a steamer, cook the asparagus spears in ½ inch simmering water in a skillet or saucepan.

Tip: Use whole-wheat English muffins for even more nutrients.

Note: Eggs Benedict and Asparagus is a prime example of a special breakfast or brunch you might prepare on a leisurely weekend morning. Note that, with the asparagus and orange juice, you've already started the day with two servings of fruits and vegetables.

Source: Healthy Heart Cookbook For Dummies

Pancetta and Spinach Frittata

Prep time: 5 min • **Cook time:** 35 min • **Yield:** 4 servings

Ingredients	Directions
Nonstick cooking spray	*1* Preheat the oven to 325 degrees. In a heavy, oven-proof skillet (preferably cast iron), heat 1 tablespoon of the olive oil over medium heat.
1 tablespoon plus 2 teaspoons olive oil	
¼ pancetta, diced small	*2* Add in the pancetta and cook for 3 to 5 minutes, until crispy. add the garlic and cook for 30 seconds. Add the spinach and sauté for 4 minutes or until lightly wilted. Strain the mixture to remove excess liquid.
2 cloves garlic, crushed	
8 cups baby spinach, rinsed and patted dry	
6 eggs, lightly beaten	*3* Heat the remaining olive oil over medium-high heat. Return the vegetable mixture to the skillet and sauté for 1 minute. Spread the vegetables evenly in a layer at the bottom of the pan.
¼ teaspoon salt	
¼ teaspoon pepper	
2 ounces feta, crumbled	*4* Add the eggs and season with the salt and pepper. Gently stir for about a minute. Let the pan sit over low heat for a minute or two or until the mixture begins to set, getting firm in the center.
	5 Top with the cheese and transfer to the oven. Bake for 10 to 12 minutes or until the eggs are set. Remove the pan from the oven and let the mixture rest for 3 minutes.
	6 Transfer the frittata to a cutting board, slice into four pie wedges, and serve hot or at room temperature.

Per serving: Calories 256 (From fat 196); Total fat 22 g (Saturated 7 g); Protein 12 g; Carbohydrate 4 g (Dietary fiber 1 g); Cholesterol 32 mg; Sodium 670 mg.

Vary It! In place of pancetta, you can substitute bacon or Canadian bacon; you get a similar taste while using up any meats you have on hand. For a vegetarian breakfast, simply omit the meat.

Source: Mediterranean Diet Cookbook For Dummies

Orange Ricotta Pancakes

Prep time: 10 min • **Cook time:** 15 min • **Yield:** 6 servings

Ingredients	Directions
1½ cups flour	*1* In a medium bowl, combine the flour, baking powder, and salt until well blended.
1 teaspoon baking powder	
½ teaspoon salt	
3 eggs, separated	*2* In a large bowl, whisk together the egg yolks, milk, ricotta, sugar, vanilla and orange zest. Add the egg yolk mixture to the dry ingredients, mix well, and set aside.
1¾ cups milk	
6 ounces low-fat ricotta cheese	*3* Using an electric mixer, beat the egg whites on medium-high speed until frothy and then turn the speed up to high until soft peaks form. Fold the egg white mixture into the batter.
¼ cup sugar	
1 tablespoon vanilla extract	
2 tablespoons fresh orange zest	*4* Spray a griddle or large nonstick skillet with nonstick cooking spray. Heat the pan over medium heat.
Nonstick cooking spray	*5* Pour ¼ cup of the batter onto the pan, evenly spacing as many pancakes as you can fit. When bubbles begin to form, flip and allow the pancakes to finish cooking, about 1 to 2 minutes. Transfer the cooked pancakes to a plate and continue cooking the remaining batter.
½ cup orange marmalade	
2 tablespoons butter	
	6 Meanwhile, melt the orange marmalade and butter in a small pot over medium-low heat, stirring frequently until they're combined and the sauce is warm. Remove from the heat. Serve the pancakes with about one tablespoon of the orange sauce per serving.

Per serving: Calories 291 (From fat 64); Total fat 7 g (Saturated 4 g); Protein 11 g; Carbohydrate 47 g (Dietary fiber 1 g); Cholesterol 23 mg; Sodium 412 mg.

Tip: Though not in the original recipe, here's a healthy heart tip for a totally fruit-based syrup (no sugar): In a small saucepan, mash 1 large or 2 medium ripe bananas, add about ½ to ¾ cup of orange juice. Stir well. Bring to boil over medium heat and reduce mixture, stirring frequently, until syrup has the consistency you like. It usually takes only 2 or 3 minutes. Add a dash of cinnamon, stir, and serve.

Source: Mediterranean Diet Cookbook For Dummies

Chapter 17

Heart-Healthy Lunches

Workday lunches can be a challenge to heart-healthy eating. For most American adults, lunch contributes about 25 percent of daily calories, but a substantial portion of these lunchtime calories may not be the most nutrient-rich. It's so easy to bring a sandwich and chips from home or grab a combo meal at a quick serve restaurant. Research data suggests that on average eating lunch away from home adds about 158 calories to any given day's energy intake. It also results in a lower Healthy Eating Index score. On the other hand, about 20 percent of American adults skip lunch and thus miss the opportunity to consume more healthful foods.

If you find yourself in one of these situations or stuck in a rut when it comes to lunch selections, the recipes in this chapter should help. These recipes represent different flavors and textures to tempt your taste buds. You can put some together quickly on the night before. Others may be quick to prepare but take a little longer to cook. (Slow cooker tips can help here.) Most of the recipes provide multiple portions that are easily refrigerated or frozen to provide more than one microwavable lunch.

Heart-healthy fruits, vegetables, legumes, and whole grains take center stage in these salads and soups. A hearty chili and a picadillo round out these versatile dishes. I've thrown in a special treat that takes a little more preparation but may be just right for a weekend lunch or an office celebration.

What? No Sandwiches?

You probably have the sandwich drill down already. Nevertheless, here are few reminders of how to pack healthy nutrients into your sandwiches:

🖊 Select a wholegrain or true sourdough bread or roll.

🖊 Make your protein lean. Good choices include lean ham, turkey, or light tuna (packed in water), low-fat cheese, hummus (from chickpeas or other legume), or a hardboiled egg.

🖊 Add lots of vegetables, such as lettuce, mixed greens, spinach, tomato, cucumber, green or red bell peppers, and grated carrot or radish to your sandwich.

🖊 Dress the sandwich with mustard rather than mayo. Or use oil and vinegar or vinaigrette — drizzle a little on the vegetables to keep the sandwich from getting soggy.

You can use these tips whether you make your sandwich at home or order it at a deli or restaurant.

Salads That Go beyond Green

Salads have long been a brown-bag lunch favorite. But green salad every day quickly gets boring. Here are four salads that feature legumes or grains, which help keep you satisfied all afternoon. Plus these recipes also include plenty of antioxidant- and vitamin-rich vegetables, as well as heart-healthy olive oil.

What vegetables, fruits, and grains do you like or do you want to try? Using these recipes as models, experiment with creating your own salads. For example, you might try simple substitutions: replacing couscous with quinoa or brown rice, for example, or trying white beans instead of black beans or chickpeas. Then you can try different combinations of vegetables and fruits. And if you make a mistake? Don't worry. Try again.

Curried Israeli Couscous Salad

Prep time: 10 min • **Cook time:** 13 min • **Yield:** 12 servings

Ingredients	Directions
2 cups Israeli couscous (or Middle Eastern couscous)	**1** In a medium saucepan, bring the water to a boil.
5 cups water	**2** Add the couscous and let the water come to a boil again. Simmer uncovered for 2 to 3 minutes.
2 teaspoons curry powder	
⅓ cup extra virgin olive oil	**3** Remove the couscous from the heat, cover, and let stand 8 to 10 minutes.
¾ cup grated carrots	
¾ cup raisins	**4** Transfer the couscous into a strainer and rinse under running water. Drain thoroughly, and then transfer to a medium-sized mixing bowl.
⅓ cup chopped cilantro, loosely packed	
Salt to taste	**5** In a small bowl, mix the curry powder and olive oil.
	6 Stir the curry-oil mixture into the couscous.
	7 Add the remaining ingredients, toss well, and season to taste with salt.

Per serving: Calories 195 (From fat 54); Total fat 6 g (Saturated 1 g); Protein 4 g; Carbohydrate 31 g (Dietary fiber 2 g); Cholesterol 0 mg; Sodium 8 mg.

Source: Healthy Heart Cookbook For Dummies

What is couscous?

Couscous is a traditional grain dish of north Africa and the Middle East. It is traditionally made of semolina (hard Durum wheat flour). The granules may be small, as in Middle Eastern couscous, or pearl size, as in Israeli couscous.

Sardinian couscous is pearl size and toasted to give a slightly nutty flavor. Whole wheat couscous is also available and has a nutty flavor. You can find Israeli couscous in specialty or ethnic stores or online. Try all types for variety.

Citrus Quinoa Salad

Prep time: 30 min • **Yield:** 8 servings

Ingredients	Directions

Ingredients

1½ cups chicken stock (vegetable stock can be substituted)

¾ cup quinoa, washed and rinsed well

¼ cup finely diced red onion

¼ cup finely diced carrot

¼ cup finely diced radish

3 to 4 scallions (green onions), washed and diagonally sliced ¼ inch thick

Salad dressing (see the recipe that follows)

Directions

1 In a medium saucepan, bring chicken stock to a boil. Add the quinoa and cook over low heat until the liquid is absorbed and the quinoa is tender, about 15 minutes.

2 Prep all the salad vegetables while the quinoa is cooking.

3 When the quinoa is fully cooked, remove it from the heat and strain it; then cool it by spreading it out on a cookie sheet as you prepare the salad dressing.

4 In a large bowl, combine all the vegetables with the cooled quinoa and toss with the dressing. Season to taste with salt and pepper.

Salad Dressing

Zest of 1 orange

¼ orange, peeled and minced

Zest of 1 lemon

¼ lemon, peeled and minced

1 tablespoon fresh lemon juice

1½ teaspoons fresh garlic, minced

1 tablespoon citrus oil or canola oil

1 tablespoon extra virgin olive oil

1½ teaspoons rice wine vinegar

1 tablespoon parsley, finely chopped

Salt and freshly ground pepper, to taste

1 Zest the orange and lemon by finely grating the outer layer of peel. Be sure to wash the fruit prior to zesting.

2 Combine all salad dressing ingredients in small bowl and season with salt and pepper.

Per serving (salad with dressing): *Calories 107 (from fat 40); Total fat 5 g (Saturated 0;5 g), Protein 3 g; Carbohydrate 14 g (Dietary fiber 2 g); Cholesterol 0 mg; Sodium 199 mg (Sodium information based on no added salt)*

Source: Healthy Heart Cookbook For Dummies

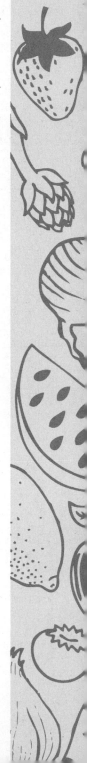

Chickpea Salad

Prep time: 20 min • **Cook time:** 5 min • **Yield:** 6 servings

Ingredients	Directions
1 cup chicken or vegetable broth	*1* In a small saucepan, bring the broth to a boil over high heat. Add the barley, cover, and remove the pot from the heat to rest for 15 minutes.
½ cup pearl barley	
One 15-ounce can chickpeas, rinsed and drained	*2* Meanwhile, combine the chickpeas, apricots, onion, parsley, lemon zest and juice, olive oil, and spices in a bowl.
1 cup diced apricots	
1 small red onion, thinly sliced	*3* Add the cooked barley and stir to mix well. Add the hot sauce and sea salt to taste.
1 cup parsley, chopped and stems discarded	
Zest and juice of 2 lemons	*4* Place the baby spinach leaves on a serving platter and spoon the warmed chickpea/barley mixture over the top. Top the salad with the pistachios and serve.
¼ cup olive oil	
¼ teaspoon pepper	
¼ teaspoon cardamom	
⅛ teaspoon ginger	
⅛ teaspoon cinnamon	
¼ teaspoon turmeric	
Dash of hot sauce	
Sea salt to taste	
8 cups baby spinach leaves	
1 cup shelled pistachios	

Per serving: Calories 368 (From fat 184); Total fat 20 g (Saturated 3 g); Protein 12 g; Carbohydrate 39 g (Dietary fiber 8 g); Cholesterol 0 mg; Sodium 580 mg.

Tip: Although not suggested in the original recipe, if this recipe makes more than you need for one meal, refrigerate the chickpea/barley mixture for a day and be ready to take it for lunch the next day. Package the chickpea/barley mixture in a separate container from the spinach and pistachios. Keep both containers refrigerated until lunchtime; then warm the chickpea mixture in the microwave and spoon over the top of your spinach and pistachios.

Source: Mediterranean Diet Cookbook For Dummies

Black Beans with Tomatoes and Feta

Prep time: 10 min • **Yield:** 8 servings

Ingredients	Directions
4 Roma or plum tomatoes, diced	**1** In a serving bowl, toss together everything but the feta and salt.
Two 14.5-ounce cans black beans, drained and rinsed	**2** Before serving, top the mixture with the feta and season with salt to taste.
½ red onion, sliced	
¼ cup fresh dill, chopped	
Juice of 1 lemon	
2 tablespoons extra-virgin olive oil	
¼ cup crumbled feta cheese	
Salt to taste	

Per serving: Calories 121 (From fat 42); Total fat 5 g (Saturated 1 g); Protein 6 g; Carbohydrate 15 g (Dietary fiber 5 g); Cholesterol 4 mg; Sodium 173 mg.

Vary It! You can substitute fresh basil for the dill for a sweet flavor.

Tip: Though this suggestion isn't with the original recipe, you can easily halve this recipe to create two lunch servings of 1 cup. Serve the bean salad with mixed greens and a slice of crusty sourdough bread for a complete lunch that's pretty to look at and delicious to eat.

Source: Mediterranean Diet Cookbook For Dummies

More about feta cheese

In Greece, feta is the most popular cheese, and it used widely in other Mediterranean countries, as well as in the rest of Europe and in North America. Traditional feta is a white cheese that is made of sheep milk or a combination of sheep and goat milk. Feta-type cheese is also prepared, particularly in the U.S., from cow milk. It is made from brined curds and has no skin. It typically comes packaged in blocks or crumbles in brine. Firm feta is tangier than soft feta, which is more spreadable.

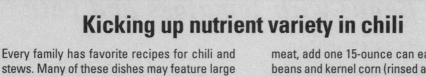

Kicking up nutrient variety in chili

Every family has favorite recipes for chili and stews. Many of these dishes may feature large portions of meat. One way to up your intake of vegetables is to add them to these dishes. Here are some ideas that may work for you:

✔ Beans are a natural partner for chili. Make a three-bean chili by adding one 15-ounce can each of pinto, red, and great northern beans (rinsed and drained) to 1 pound of ground meat. You can also add 1 cup of diced carrots.

✔ Add black beans, corn, and pimentos to make a "fiesta" chili. For each pound of meat, add one 15-ounce can each of black beans and kernel corn (rinsed and drained), and one small jar of pimentos (drained).

✔ Turn your favorite ground meat chili recipe into a tasty sauce for pasta by adding one 15-ounce can of diced tomatoes and 1 cup diced carrots. Cook until the carrots are soft and the liquid reduces to the appropriate consistency for sauce. Ten minutes before serving, add 1 cup chopped broccoli, 1 cup fresh asparagus (cut in 2-inch lengths), or 2 cups of broccoli flowerets.

Soups, Chili, and Picadillo

Soups and chili appeal particularly in cooler weather, but these recipes are good all year long. You'll feel like you've taken a mini international gourmet tour if you try them all — no jaded palate here.

Although most of these recipes take about an hour to cook, you can easily make them the night before; most can be made in a slow cooker.

Each recipe provides multiple servings. Consider refrigerating the leftovers or freezing them in meal-sized portions, giving you several quick, healthy lunches. You can do the same with your family's favorite soup, chili, and stew recipes.

Spicy African Chicken Soup

Prep time: 30 min • **Cook time:** 60 min • **Yield:** Sixteen 1-cup servings

Ingredients	Directions
2 tablespoons olive oil	**1** In a large saucepan, heat the olive oil over low heat. Add the onions, celery, and garlic, and cook, stirring often until soft.
1½ cups diced onion	
1 cup chopped celery	
5 teaspoons minced garlic	**2** Add the chicken stock, tomatoes, parsley, cinnamon stick, cloves, bay leaves, and cayenne pepper. Increase heat to bring the soup to a slow boil.
8 cups (64 fluid ounces) chicken stock	
3½ cups (28 fluid ounces) canned tomatoes, diced, with juice	**3** Reduce the heat to low; simmer for 20 minutes, stirring occasionally.
½ cup + 1 tablespoon minced parsley	**4** Add the bulgur wheat and the chicken and continue to simmer for 15 minutes.
½ cinnamon stick	
Pinch ground cloves (about ¼ teaspoon)	**5** Remove the cinnamon stick and bay leaves. Season to taste with salt and pepper.
2 bay leaves	
Pinch cayenne pepper (about ¼ teaspoon)	**6** Ladle the soup into soup bowls. Top with unsalted, dry roasted peanuts (optional).
2 cups uncooked bulgur wheat	
12 ounces chicken breast (without skin) cut into strips approximately 1½ inches long and ½ inch thick	
2 teaspoons salt (omit if using chicken broth with sodium)	
1 teaspoon coarsely ground black pepper (use more to add spiciness)	

Per serving: Calories 111 (From fat 27); Total fat 3 g (Saturated 0.7 g); Protein 9 g; Carbohydrate 12 g (Dietary fiber 3 g); Cholesterol 13 mg; Sodium 620 mg.

Tip: Extra soup may be refrigerated for two to three days or frozen for two months.

Source: Heart Disease For Dummies

Pumpkin Soup

Prep time: 25 min • **Cook time:** 1 hr, 15 min • **Yield:** 8 servings

Ingredients	Directions
1 small (2½ to 3 pound) pumpkin, peeled, seeded, and cut into 2-inch chunks	*1* Preheat oven to 400 degrees.
2 large onions, coarsely chopped	*2* Combine the pumpkin, onions, garlic, potatoes, rosemary, and olive oil in a large bowl and toss to coat evenly.
6 cloves fresh garlic	
2 large potatoes, peeled and cut into 1-inch cubes	*3* Roast the vegetables for 50 minutes or until the vegetables are lightly brown and somewhat tender.
4 large sprigs fresh rosemary	*4* Transfer the roasted vegetables to a soup pot.
2 tablespoons olive oil	
8 cups vegetable stock	*5* Cover with vegetable stock, stir and bring to a boil. Lower temperature and simmer and cook until flavors blend, about 20 to 30 minutes.
1 bunch fresh thyme	
Salt and pepper, to taste	
	6 Puree the mixture in batches (enough to half fill your blender or food processor bowl) in blender or food processor. Return the mixture to the soup pot to keep warm and season with salt and pepper to taste. Serve warm.

Per serving: Calories 136 (From fat 36); Total fat 4 g (Saturated 1 g); Protein 3 g; Carbohydrate 25 g (Dietary fiber 5 g); Cholesterol 0 mg; Sodium 997 mg.

Tip: No pumpkin in the supermarket? Substitute another orange-fleshed winter squash such as butternut, buttercup, delicata, kabocha, or kuri. You can also substitute canned or frozen pumpkin. Simply add it to the soup pot with the roasted vegetables in Step 4.

Source: Healthy Heart Cookbook For Dummies

Lentil Soup with Tomatoes and Spinach

Prep time: 8 min • **Cook time:** 45 min • **Yield:** 8 servings

Ingredients	Directions
1 tablespoon olive oil	**1** Heat the olive oil into a large stock pot over medium heat. After 1 minute, add the onions, carrot, and celery and cook until the onions are translucent, about 6 to 7 minutes.
1 cup chopped onion	
½ cup carrot, diced small	
½ cup celery, diced small	
1½ teaspoon salt	**2** Add the salt, lentils, tomatoes, broth, coriander, cumin, and bay leaf and stir to combine. Increase the heat to high and bring just to a boil.
1 pound orange or brown lentils	
One 14.5-ounce can unsalted chopped tomatoes	**3** Reduce the heat to low, cover, and cook at a low simmer until the lentils are tender, about 35 to 40 minutes. Add the spinach in the last 15 minutes or simply add to each bowl for serving. Season with salt and pepper to taste and serve immediately.
8 cups chicken or vegetable broth	
½ teaspoon ground coriander	
½ teaspoon ground cumin	
1 bay leaf	
5 ounces baby spinach leaves	
Salt and pepper to taste	

Per serving: Calories 285 (From fat 35); Total fat 4 g (Saturated 1 g); Protein 21 g; Carbohydrate 42 g (Dietary fiber 19 g); Cholesterol 0 mg; Sodium 959 mg.

Tip: To use a slow cooker, combine all the ingredients except the spinach in the slow cooker and cook for 6 hours on low. Add the spinach during the last 15 minutes of cooking or to each bowl for serving.

Source: Mediterranean Diet Cookbook For Dummies

Picadillo

Prep time: 15 min • **Cook time:** 60 min • **Yield:** Eight 1½ cup servings

Ingredients	Directions

Ingredients

1 pound ground pork, lamb, or beef (analysis based on using ground pork)

1 yellow onion, peeled and finely chopped

3 cloves garlic, peeled and minced

5 carrots, peeled and shredded

1 green pepper, seeded and coarsely chopped

½ small head of green cabbage, finely chopped

1 teaspoon dried oregano (or 1 tablespoon fresh)

1 teaspoon dried thyme (or 1 tablespoon fresh)

2 bay leaves

2½ cups water

One 28-ounce can tomato puree

One 28-ounce can of whole tomatoes

1 tablespoon soy sauce

2 tablespoons red wine or dry sherry

1 cup uncooked rice

Salt and pepper to taste

Directions

1 Brown the ground meat in a sauté pan or skillet over medium-high heat. After about 5 minutes, when the meat is fully cooked, transfer to a strainer and drain thoroughly over a bowl. Discard drained fat and liquid. Press meat between several thicknesses of paper towels to remove excess fat.

2 Place meat in a 3-quart saucepan over medium heat. Add the chopped onions and garlic and sauté for 5 minutes.

3 Add the remaining ingredients, stir, cover, and bring to a boil. Reduce heat and simmer for 45 minutes. Stir occasionally to prevent sticking or burning on the bottom.

4 Serve with warmed corn tortillas and your favorite beverage.

Per serving: Calories 270 (From fat 32); Total fat 3.5 g (Saturated 1 g); Protein 18 g; Carbohydrate 43 g (Dietary fiber 6 g); Cholesterol 32 mg; Sodium 706 mg.

Note: Picadillo (pronounced pee-kah-DEE-yoh) is a common dish in many Spanish-speaking countries, but it's universally appealing. The name comes from the Spanish word for *chop* and refers to a meat stew or hash. Different regional picadillo recipes will have different ingredients, but this one works great in American kitchens.

Tip: It's easy to pack picadillo for lunch in a microwavable container. Why not freeze individual servings in ready-to-go microwavable containers. Individual servings of corn tortillas wrapped in airtight plastic wrap and baggies will also freeze easily for two weeks or so.

Source: Healthy Heart Cookbook For Dummies

Spicy Vegetarian Pinto Bean Chili

Prep time: 20 min • **Cook time:** 1 hr, 20 min • **Yield:** 8 servings

Ingredients	Directions
2 tablespoons canola oil	**1** Heat the canola oil over medium-high heat in a large stockpot, soup pot, or Dutch oven. Add the chopped onions and garlic and sauté for 2 to 3 minutes.
1 medium onion, finely chopped	
4 cloves garlic, finely chopped	**2** Add the red pepper flakes, jalapeno, green and red peppers, celery, and carrots, and continue cooking, stirring often, for another 1 to 2 minutes.
1 tablespoon red pepper flakes	
2 jalapeno peppers, seed, cored, and diced	**3** Add the crushed tomatoes and stir well.
1 large green bell pepper, seeded, cored, and chopped	**4** Add the remaining ingredients.
1 large red bell pepper, seeded, cored, and chopped	**5** Stir again, cover, reduce heat to low, and allow the soup to simmer for at least 1 hour. Stir occasionally to prevent sticking or burning.
4 stalks celery, trimmed and sliced crosswise	
4 carrots, peeled and grated	**6** Serve warm. Be sure to remove the bay leaf before serving.
One 28-ounce can crushed tomatoes	
One 12-ounce can tomato paste	**7** Refrigerate extra chili for up to four days or freeze.
3½ cups water	
6 cups cooked pinto beans (or canned, drained and rinsed beans)	
One 15½ –ounce can whole kernel corn, drained and rinsed	
1 teaspoon pepper	
½ teaspoon salt	
1½ teaspoons dried oregano	
2 teaspoons sugar	
1 bay leaf	

Per serving: Calories 351 (From fat 40); Total fat 5 g (Saturated, less than 1 g); Protein 6 g; Carbohydrate 67 g (Dietary fiber 18 g); Cholesterol 0 mg; Sodium 987 mg.

Vary It! If you don't love spicy food, you can make this chili with less heat. Just leave out the pepper flakes and jalapenos or adjust the quantity to your taste. You can also add a teaspoon each of ground cumin and sweet or smoked paprika to boost the chili flavor. Top with a couple of tablespoons of low fat cheddar or jack cheese for extra flavor (cheese not included in nutritional facts).

Vary It! Experiment with different combinations of beans for different flavors and textures. Try 1 can each of pintos, red beans, and great northern, drained and rinsed, for example, or 1 can each of black beans, navy beans, cranberry beans, drained and rinsed. (Draining and rinsing reduces the sodium in canned beans.)

Tip: You can use a slow cooker prepare this chili: To do so, follow the recipe through Step 4, and then place the mixture in a slow cooker. If you plan to take the chili to work for lunch the next day, cook it overnight (about 6 hours) on low and then pack up lunch containers and refrigerate the rest. If you plan to eat the chili for dinner that night, place the lid on the slow cooker bowl and refrigerate. In the morning, place the bowl in the slow cooker and let it cook all day on low while you are at work.

Tip: This chili makes a great one-dish lunch. Store single servings in microwave-safe containers, store in the refrigerator at work, and microwave until heated throughout. Also, serve it for dinner with a green salad and corn muffins.

Source: Healthy Heart Cookbook For Dummies

Make your own chili powder

Do you ever get tired of making chili using the prepared chili powders you find in the supermarket? Then make your own. The Spicy Vegetarian Pinto Bean Chili recipe, as you'll notice, doesn't use chili powder but has red pepper flakes, jalapenos, garlic, and oregano, which are typical ingredients found in many chili powders.

When you make your own chili powder, you can vary the flavor and heat to suit your taste and the dish you are making. For a chili pepper foundation choose from sweet paprika, Hungarian paprika, smoked paprika, ground ancho chile (dried poblano pepper), cayenne pepper, and ground chipotle chiles (dried jalapeños). Then select from such additional spices as garlic powder, ground cumin, and ground oregano or Mexican oregano. When you arrive at a combination you like, store the mixture in an airtight container.

One final hint: Make your trial with small amounts — teaspoons and fractions of teaspoons — until you get the right balance.

A Leisurely or Celebratory Lunch

Here's a dish that is great for a weekend lunch or for appetizers at a party. Until you've done it a few times, preparing the ingredients takes a little time, but the results are worth the effort. It's also fun to mix cultural styles and serve these rolls with Spicy White Bean Dip (you can find that recipe in Chapter 19) and raw vegetable chunks for dipping. Make the Citrus Tea first to enjoy as you prepare the meal and then to accompany it.

Citrus Tea

Prep time: 60 min, including chill time • **Cook time:** 5 min • **Yield:** 4 servings

Ingredients	Directions
Juice from 2 limes	**1** Combine the lime juice, orange juice, water, lemon grass, herb tea, and sugar in a medium saucepan and bring to a boil over high heat.
Juice from 1 orange	
4 cups water	
1 stalk chopped lemon grass	**2** Once boiling, turn off the heat and let the tea sit on the burner for 5 minutes.
4 bags orange-flavored herb tea	
1 tablespoons sugar	**3** Pour the tea mixture through a strainer, place the strained tea in a large pitcher, and chill in refrigerator for about an hour.
Lemon, lime or orange slices, for garnish (optional)	
	4 When chilled, pour over ice and serve in glasses garnished with lemon, lime, or orange slices.

Per serving: Calories 36 (From fat 0); Total fat 0 g (Saturated 0 g); Protein 0 g; Carbohydrate 9 g (Dietary fiber 0 g); Cholesterol 0 mg; Sodium 6 mg.

Source: Healthy Heart Cookbook For Dummies

Rice Vermicelli and Salad Rolls with Peanut Sauce

Prep time: 20–30 min • **Cook time:** 3 min • **Yield:** 8 servings (1 roll plus sauce)

Ingredients	Directions
2 ounces uncooked rice vermicelli noodles **1 large carrot, peeled and shredded** **1 tablespoon sugar** **1 tablespoon fish sauce** **Eight 8-inch round rice paper sheets** **8 large romaine or iceberg lettuce leaves, washed, thick stalks removed** **12 ounces roast pork, thinly sliced** **4 ounces (approximately 1 $\frac{2}{3}$ cups) bean sprouts** **Handful (about 16) mint leaves** **8 cooked king prawns (or jumbo shrimp), peeled, deveined and halved lengthwise** **½ cucumber, cut into fine strips (julienned)** **Cilantro leaves, for garnish** **Peanut Sauce (see the following recipe)**	**1** Soak the rice vermicelli in a large bowl filled with warm water until the noodles soften. **2** While the vermicelli noodles are soaking, fill a large saucepan with water and bring to a boil. When the water is boiling and the noodles have softened, drop the noodles into the boiling water and cook for 1 to 2 minutes or just until the noodles are tender and lose their raw taste. **3** Drain the noodles, rinse them under cold running water, and drain again. **4** In a medium bowl, combine the vermicelli, carrots, sugar, and fish sauce. Toss well. **5** Dip one of the rice sheets in a bowl of warm water, and then lay it flat on the table or countertop. On the rice sheet, place 1 lettuce leaf, 1 to 2 scoops of the noodle mixture, a few slices of roast pork, some of the bean sprouts, and 2 mint leaves. Keep in mind that all filling ingredients need to be divided into 8 servings — try not to shortchange the person who will get the eighth roll! **6** Start rolling up the rice sheet into a cylinder. When half the sheet has been rolled up, fold both sides of the sheet toward the center and lay two prawn (or shrimp) halves along the crease. **7** Add a few strips of cucumber and some cilantro. Continue to roll up the sheet to make a tight packet. Place the roll on a large serving plate and cover with a damp dishtowel to keep the roll moist while you assemble the rest of the rolls.

8 Repeat Steps 5 through 7 until all the rolls have been assembled.

9 To serve, cut each roll in half. Serve with 2 tablespoons of the Peanut Sauce.

Peanut Sauce

1 tablespoon canola oil

3 cloves garlic, peeled and finely chopped

1 to 2 red chili peppers, seeded and finely chopped

1 teaspoon tomato puree

½ cup water

1 tablespoon creamy peanut butter (preferably freshly ground peanut butter)

2 tablespoons hoisin sauce

½ teaspoon sugar

Juice of 1 lime

2 ounces (approximately 6 tablespoons) roasted, unsalted peanuts, finely chopped or ground

1 In a small saucepan over high heat, heat the oil. Add the garlic, chili peppers, and tomato puree and cook for 1 minute, stirring continuously.

2 Add the water and bring to a boil.

3 Stir in peanut butter, hoisin sauce, sugar, and fresh lime juice. Mix well.

4 Reduce heat and simmer for 3 to 4 minutes.

5 Transfer the sauce into a small serving bowl, top with the ground peanuts, and allow to cool to room temperature before serving.

Per serving for the rolls: Calories 183 (From fat 54); Total fat 6 g (Saturated 2 g); Protein 17 g; Carbohydrate 16 g (Dietary fiber 1 g); Cholesterol 47 mg; Sodium 108 mg.

Per serving for peanut sauce: Calories 86 (From fat 63); Total fat 7 g (Saturated 1 g); Protein 3 g; Carbohydrate 5 g (Dietary fiber 1 g); Cholesterol 0 mg; Sodium 111 mg.

Tip: These rolls take a little effort to make, but they are delicious. Two make a terrific light lunch. The rice paper sheets can be so fragile that it takes a little practice to wrap them without splitting the sheet, but they eat really well with a fork!

Source: Healthy Heart Cookbook For Dummies

Chapter 18

Heart-Healthy Dinners

In This Chapter

▶ Preparing ahead for quick and easy dinners

▶ Grilling entrees any time of year

▶ Making vegetarian and meat-based main dishes

Sitting down together to a home-cooked meal at dinner is a challenge for busy families. Work schedules for parents and school activities for children can make it hard to find the time to fix dinner, much less sit down together to eat. That's one reason, no doubt, that a great percentage of the money spent on food in the U.S. goes to take-out and restaurant meals.

Eating together as a family (see Chapter 7) and eating a healthful meal at home, however, both contribute to better overall health and heart health. It's also a time to share as a family and strengthen family connections and support. With that in mind, this chapter offers recipes for dinner meals or main dishes that you can fix ahead or fix quickly. Other recipes may be more suitable to a weekend or vacation day.

TIP

A few may seem to have a long list of ingredients and preparation steps, but if you look more closely at the recipe, you'll see that in most cases the ingredients are for quickly prepared marinades or sauces that accompany the main dish. Most can be used for more than one meal or dish and are easy to refrigerate or freeze for later use. Flexibility is the key concept to keep in mind as you think about making these recipes part of your regular meal planning.

But what if you are one of the 32 million American adults who live alone? All the recipes seem to have four to eight servings. Well, you are about to be in the winner's seat. You can invite friends over or cut a recipe in half, or you can make the whole recipe, enjoy one dinner, refrigerate one for later in the week, and freeze individual portions for later meals that are typically more delicious and nutritious (not to mention less costly) than take-out or restaurant meals.

Easy Fix-Ahead Dinners

All the meals in this section taste great when fixed ahead. With the Ratatouille and Pot-au-Feu of Chicken, chopping up the vegetables may take the most time, but you can prepare these meals in two steps: Prep the vegetables one night and cook the dish the next.

The Chili Lime Game Hens with Cranberry Pecan Salsa also makes the fix-ahead list because you can marinate the game hens (or chicken breasts or quarters) overnight. And you can easily double the salsa recipe to use for other dishes.

Although fix-ahead dishes make meal preparation faster and easier, many people find even that hard to squeeze into family members' busy schedules. In that case, three tips may make pre-preparation easier:

- **Divide the load.** Mom isn't the only one who can cook. As I discuss in Chapter 7, involving all family members in meal planning and preparation helps children try a greater variety of foods and helps older kids and adults buy into family meals.

- **Put fix-ahead time on your schedules.** Once every week or two weeks, decide who will fix a dish ahead and when. Write it down or enter it on individual calendars.

- **Spark interest in meals with a new menu chart.** Research shows that most families eat the same 10 meals over and over. The result? Boredom. A good way to use old and new recipes (like those in this book) is to sit down with the family and the cookbooks and magazines with recipes you want to try. Make up a chart with 30 dinner menus; note where any new recipes are found. Family members responsible for cooking can then pick a menu each would like to try and plan and prepare ahead.

Pot-au-Feu of Chicken

Prep time: 2 hrs • **Cook time:** 1 hr, 15 min • **Yield:** 4 servings

Ingredients	Directions
1 small whole chicken (2½ to 3 pounds), trimmed and cleaned with cold water; skin removed	**1** Place the chicken in a 4-quart soup or stock pot, cover with cold water, and bring to a boil. Reduce heat to simmer.
1 teaspoon salt	
2 bay leaves	**2** Add the salt, bay leaves, thyme, garlic, carrots, onions, celery, parsnips, leek, cabbage, fennel, and potatoes. Simmer over low heat for 1 hour, skimming the surface as necessary until the chicken is tender and cooked through. Add the peas during the last 3 minutes of cooking.
1 teaspoon fresh thyme, or ½ teaspoon dried	
6 cloves fresh garlic	
2 carrots, peeled and cut into 1-inch pieces	
6 pearl onions, peeled	**3** Place four soup plates in a warm oven to preheat for 2 to 3 minutes. Using kitchen tongs or a carving fork, carefully lift the chicken out of the pot, draining any liquid in the cavity back into the soup pot. Transfer the chicken to a large cutting board and carve so that each diner receives half of a breast and half of a leg. Divide the chicken among four preheated soup plates, and ladle the broth and vegetables over the chicken.
2 stalks of celery, cut into 1-inch pieces	
2 parsnips, peeled and cut into 1-inch pieces	
1 leek, root end trimmed, halved lengthwise, thoroughly washed, white and light green part cut into 1-inch pieces	
½ head of green cabbage, cut into 4 wedges	**4** Sprinkle with parsley and serve.
1 fennel bulb, quartered	
2 medium red-skinned potatoes, quartered	
½ cup fresh or frozen green peas	
2 tablespoons chopped fresh parsley, for garnish	

Per serving: Calories 381 (From fat 72); Total fat 8 g (Saturated 2 g); Protein 35 g; Carbohydrate 45 g (Dietary fiber 11 g); Cholesterol 87 mg; Sodium 782 mg.

Source: Healthy Heart Cookbook For Dummies

Ratatouille

Prep time: 30 min • **Cook time:** 1 hr, 30 min • **Yield:** 6 servings

Ingredients	Directions
2 tablespoons olive oil	*1* Preheat oven to 300 degrees.
2 pounds (3 to 4 small) egg-plants, ends trimmed, cut into 1-inch cubes	*2* Heat the oil in a medium heavy-bottom saucepan over medium-high heat. Add the eggplant, onions, garlic, peppers, and zucchini, and sauté, stirring often, for 5 minutes. Season with salt and add the tomatoes, tomato paste, and bay leaf. Bring to a simmer.
2 large onions, sliced	
6 large cloves garlic (4 cloves sliced or minced and 2 cloves put through a press or pureed)	
1 large red bell pepper, cut into slices about 1 inch wide and 2 inches long	*3* In a large earthenware dish, combine the sautéed vegetables and the thyme, oregano, and coriander, and bake for about 1 hour, 20 minutes, until the vegetables are completely tender.
1 large green bell pepper, cut into slices about 1 inch wide and 2 inches long	
1½ pounds (3 medium size) zucchini, cut in half length-wise and sliced ½ inch thick	
Coarse sea salt to taste	
4 large (or 6 medium) toma-toes, peeled, seeded, and coarsely chopped	
1 tablespoon tomato paste	
1 bay leaf	

2 teaspoons fresh thyme leaves, or 1 teaspoon crushed dried thyme

1 teaspoon crushed dried oregano, or 2 teaspoons chopped fresh oregano

½ teaspoon crushed coriander seeds

Per serving: Calories 168 (From fat 53); Total fat 5.6 g (Saturated 0.8 g); Protein 5 g; Carbohydrate 28 g (Dietary fiber 8g); Cholesterol 0 mg; Sodium 43 mg (based on no added salt).

Tip: Ratatouille is one of those dishes that often tastes even better on the second day. So make it the night before, refrigerate, and reheat for dinner the next evening. It's a great vegetarian main dish. Or pair it as a side dish with a take-out rotisserie chicken.

Source: The Healthy Heart Cookbook For Dummies

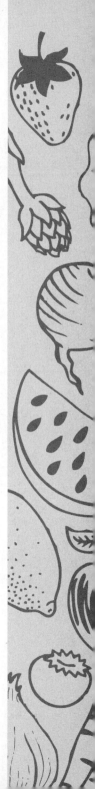

Chili Lime Game Hens with Cranberry Pecan Salsa

Prep time: 1 hr, 25 min (including marinating) • **Cook time:** 40 min • **Yield:** 4 servings

Ingredients	Directions
1 cup lime juice	**1** Combine all the ingredients except for the game hens in a blender. Blend and reserve the marinade.
½ cup olive oil	
3 tablespoons fresh chopped garlic	**2** Clean the game hens by removing the innards and rinsing the birds under cold running water. Cut out the backbone by placing the hens, breast sides down, on a cutting board. Using a sharp knife or kitchen shears, cut along both sides of the backbone for each hen. Remove the bone. Using your hands, press down to flatten the hens.
2 tablespoons ground cumin	
1 tablespoon ground cinnamon	
2 tablespoons chili powder	
2 teaspoons salt	
2 teaspoons pepper	**3** Place the hens in a deep bowl, pour the marinade mixture over them, and refrigerate for at least 1 hour.
Four 1- to 1½-pound game hens	
Cranberry Pecan Salsa (see following recipe)	**4** Preheat the oven to 375 degrees. Remove the hens from the marinade and place them on a baking sheet so that they lay flat with the skin side up.
	5 Cook uncovered for 35 to 40 minutes, until cooked through. (Cooking time varies depending on the size of each bird.)
	6 Serve each bird with ½ cup of the Cranberry Pecan Salsa.

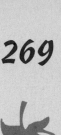

Cranberry Pecan Salsa

1 cup dried cranberries

¼ cup orange juice

¼ cup honey

1 red bell pepper, cored, seeded, and chopped

¼ cup chopped toasted pecans

¼ cup chopped cilantro

2 tablespoons lemon zest and the juice from the lemons

1 teaspoon salt

1 Combine all ingredients in a medium mixing bowl, cover, and refrigerate for at least 1 hour to allow flavors to combine.

Per serving: Calories 527 (From fat 144); total fat 16 g (Saturated 3g) (fat based on removing skin before eating); Protein 46 g; Carbohydrate 51 g (Dietary fiber 4 g); Cholesterol 202 mg; Sodium 1029 mg.

Tip: Because the salsa should be made ahead and the game hens should marinate at least an hour, this is a great recipe to prepare the evening before so that the hens can marinate overnight.

Vary It! You can easily substitute chicken breasts or chicken quarters in the recipe. Adjust cooking times as needed. Remove skin before eating.

Source: Healthy Heart Cookbook For Dummies

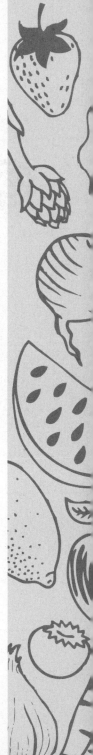

Grilling Time

Grilling out may be America's favorite way to eat in summer. But in many parts of the country, you can grill out for most of the year. When it's too cold, a stovetop grill pan or even a cast-iron skillet works very well. The first two recipes — Lime-Marinated Shrimp and Spanish Kabobs — are very easy to prepare and quick to cook. The other two — Marinated Grilled Pork Tenderloin with Raspberry Chambord Sauce and Grilled Flat Iron Steak with Chipotle Glaze Served with Wilted Escarole and Sweet Onion Salad — take more time to fix but are not hard to prepare and are great for more leisurely evenings.

Grilling tips

Grilling produces the best results when you follow the right techniques for both the grill you're using and the food you're cooking. Here are some tips to help:

✔ **Preheat the grill.** Gas, charcoal, or stovetop grills all need preheating before you start cooking.

✔ **Clean and oil the grate.** Grates on gas and charcoal grills clean best when hot. Scrape with a wire brush and then oil lightly to prevent food from sticking. Inside, use a nonstick stovetop grill. Oil as needed with lean meats and vegetables.

✔ **Use a basket for fish, vegetables, and tofu.** A grill basket makes cooking much easier for small foods or foods that tend to flake or crumble during cooking.

✔ **Use food thermometers.** To make sure meats reach a safe internal temperature, use an instant read thermometer. Beef, pork, lamb, veal, and fish should be 145 degrees Fahrenheit, ground meat 160 degrees, and chicken 165 degrees. For roasting and smoking, also use a standup or hanging thermometer within the grill to keep the heat at the desired level.

Lime-Marinated Shrimp

Prep time: 15 min, plus 1 hr for marinating • **Cook time:** 5 min • **Yield:** 4 servings

Ingredients	Directions
1 pound large to extra-large shrimp, peeled and deveined	**1** Place the shrimp in a medium mixing bowl and refrigerate.
1 cup fresh lime juice	
1 shallot, minced	**2** To another medium mixing bowl, add lime juice, shallot, garlic, chilies, scallions, cilantro, parsley, honey, and water.
2 cloves garlic, minced	
2 Serrano chilies, stemmed, seeded and finely chopped	**3** Slowly add the olive oil to the above ingredients, whisking continuously. Salt to taste.
4 scallions, thinly sliced	
½ cup cilantro, rinsed, destemmed, and finely chopped	**4** Pour the marinade over the shrimp 1 hour before grilling. Remove the shrimp from the marinade and drain 5 minutes before grilling.
½ cup parsley, rinsed, destemmed, and finely chopped	
2 tablespoons honey	**5** Place the shrimp on a clean, hot grill and cook approximately 2 minutes on each side.
½ cup water	
1 cup olive oil	**6** Season with salt and pepper to taste. Serve immediately.
Salt and pepper to taste	

Per serving: Calories 151 (From fat 36); Total fat 4 g (Saturated 1 g); Protein 18 g; Carbohydrate 10 g (Dietary fiber 0 g); Cholesterol 161 mg; Sodium 191 mg.

Tip: Make fixing these shrimp even easier by prepping the shrimp and marinade the night before. Both keep well in the refrigerator in airtight containers. Then simply drop the shrimp in the marinade when you arrive home from work. These shrimp cook particularly well on a stovetop grill pan.

Tip: Serve the Lime-Marinated Shrimp with sides of a green salad and couscous or a baked sweet or russet potato. Just cook the potatoes in the oven while the shrimp is marinating for an hour.

Source: Healthy Heart Cookbook For Dummies

Marinated Grilled Pork Tenderloin with Raspberry Chambord Sauce

Prep time: 18 min, plus 7–10 hrs for marinating • **Cook time:** 15–20 min • **Yield:** 6 servings

Ingredients	Directions
Zest and juice of one grapefruit	**1** In a large bowl, combine all the ingredients except the pork and mix with a wire whisk. Set the marinade aside.
Zest and juice of 3 limes	
Zest and juice of 2 oranges	**2** If necessary, remove all fat and the silver skin from the pork tenderloins.
6 fluid ounces (¾ cup) raspberry vinegar	
1 bunch fresh cilantro, chopped	**3** Place the trimmed tenderloins in a shallow pan and cover with the marinade.
1 cup honey	**4** Cover the pan and refrigerate for 7 to 10 hours. Make Raspberry Chambord Sauce (see the following recipe) while the meat is marinating.
3 tablespoons soy oil or canola oil	
Two 16-ounce pork tenderloins, trimmed of all fat and silver skin removed	**5** When you are ready to cook the meat, preheat the grill. Place the rack 3 to 4 inches from the heat source. When the grill is hot, grill the tenderloins, turning to brown all sides, for 10 to 12 minutes for medium or 15 to 18 minutes for medium-well to well-done. Use an instant-read meat thermometer to assure that the internal temperature has reached 150 to 165 degrees. Remove the tenderloins from the heat and let rest for 5 minutes (cooking will continue).
	6 Slice the tenderloins into 1½- to 2-inch medallions and serve with ⅓ cup Raspberry Chambord Sauce.

Raspberry Chambord Sauce

½ pound (1¾ cup) fresh raspberries

2 cups Burgundy wine

6 ounces (1 cup minus 2 tablespoons) sugar

1 Place the raspberries, wine, and sugar in medium saucepan.

2 Bring the mixture to a boil, reduce to a simmer, and simmer 1 hour. Strain seeds out with a fine sieve or strainer and serve.

Per serving: (for Grilled Tenderloin): Calories 302 (From fat 81); Total fat 9 g (Saturated 2.5 g); Protein 35 g; Carbohydrate 20 g (Dietary fiber 0 g); Cholesterol 96 mg; Sodium 74 mg.

Per serving: (for Raspberry Chambord Sauce): Calories 184 (From fat 0); Total fat 0 g (Saturated 0 g); Protein 0 g; Carbohydrate 35 g (Dietary fiber 0 g); Cholesterol 0 mg; Sodium 6 mg.

Tip: Because the pork tenderloin requires a long time to marinate, this is a great recipe to prepare the night before you plan to grill out.

Tip: The Raspberry Chambord Sauce may be made ahead and refrigerated to five to seven days.

Tip: The Raspberry Chambord Sauce goes great on other meats — and on vanilla ice cream!

Source: Healthy Heart Cookbook For Dummies

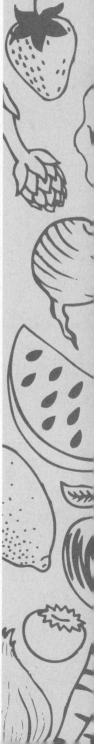

Grilled Flat Iron Steak with Chipotle Glaze Served with Wilted Escarole and Sweet Onion Salad

Prep time: 25 min • **Cook time:** 20 min • **Yield:** 4 servings

Ingredients	Directions
8 small (half-dollar size) red potatoes, rose fir or Yukon gold	*1* Place the potatoes in a saucepan with enough cold salted (optional) water to cover. Bring to a boil, reduce heat, and simmer until just tender (approximately 10 minutes).
1 medium red onion, peeled and cut into 8 wedges	*2* Coat the onion wedges with 1 tablespoon of the olive oil. Season to taste with salt (optional) and pepper.
2 tablespoons olive oil, divided	
24 ounces flat iron steak (or flank steak), trimmed and cut into 4 steaks	*3* Place the onions in a baking dish and roast for 10 minutes.
Olive oil or olive oil spray (minimal amount)	*4* Remove the onion wedges from the pan, place them on a plate, and allow them to cool to room temperature.
Kosher salt	
Pepper	*5* Drain the potatoes and allow them to cool to room temperature. When potatoes are cool, cut them in half and set aside. Do not refrigerate.
Chipotle Glaze (see following recipe)	
1 head escarole, outside leaves removed, rinsed well, and torn into small pieces	*6* Arrange the grill rack 3 to 4 inches from the heat source. Preheat your grill or stovetop grill pan.
2 teaspoons minced garlic	*7* Brush the steaks with a little olive oil; then season them with salt and pepper. When the grill is hot, place the steaks on the grill. For medium-rare, grill the steaks approximately 4 minutes on each side.
2 tablespoons balsamic vinegar	
	8 Brush the steaks with Chipotle Glaze before removing them from the grill. When they reach the desired doneness, remove the steaks from the grill and let them rest while you finish the vegetables/salad.

9   Place a large skillet over medium heat, add the remaining 1 tablespoon olive oil and heat until hot.

10   Add the cooled potatoes and cook, tossing or gently stirring occasionally, until slightly browned. Transfer the potatoes to a paper-lined plate.

11   Add the escarole and garlic to the skillet and sauté until the escarole just begins to wilt, about 2 minutes. Return the potatoes to the skillet. Add the vinegar to the escarole/potato mixture and lightly mix. Season to taste with salt and pepper.

12   Set out four dinner plates and place equal amounts of wilted escarole, potatoes, and 2 wedges of roasted onion on each serving plate.

13   Cut each portion of steak into 4 slices and arrange steak slices over the top of the greens, brush with a thin layer of Chipotle Glaze, and serve immediately.

Chipotle Glaze

1 tablespoon canned chipotle or ½ teaspoon minced, dry chipotle

2 tablespoons poblano chili peppers, minced and seeded

2 cloves garlic, peeled and minced

2 tablespoons dark molasses

1 tablespoon soy sauce

1 tablespoon dark brown sugar

1 tablespoon balsamic vinegar

2 teaspoons Dijon mustard

3 tablespoons fresh lemon juice

1 medium ripe tomato, chopped

2 cups water

¼ teaspoon kosher salt

¼ teaspoon pepper

¼ cup chopped cilantro

1 Combine all the ingredients, except the cilantro, in a 2-quart, stainless-steel heavy-bottomed saucepan. Place over high heat and bring to a boil. Reduce the heat to low and simmer for 15 to 20 minutes.

2 Remove the sauce from the heat and pour through a fine strainer. Use a wooden spoon to push through as much of the sauce as possible. Discard the solids left in the strainer.

3 Stir the cilantro into the sauce and cool completely before using.

Per serving: (based on 4 servings of salad with 2 tablespoons glaze): Calories 553 (From fat xx); Total fat 18.7 g (Saturated 5.6 g); Protein 42 g; Carbohydrate 52 g (Dietary fiber 6 g); Cholesterol 97 mg; Sodium 228 mg.

Tip: This recipe makes quite a bit more Chipotle Glaze than you need to brush the steaks. Freeze the extra servings of Chipotle Glaze in meal-size amounts (4 servings). Try the glaze on other grilled meats such as chicken or pork. The Chipotle Glaze can be stored in the refrigerator for up to four days in a tightly covered container or frozen. Reheat over low heat before serving.

Source: Healthy Heart Cookbook For Dummies

Spanish Kabobs

Prep time: 20 min, plus marinating time • **Cook time:** 16 min • **Yield:** 4 servings

Ingredients	Directions
Three 6-ounce boneless, skinless chicken breasts	*1* Cut the chicken into bite-sized pieces (about 2 inches).
¼ cup almonds	
1 teaspoon ground cumin	*2* In a food processor, pulse the almonds, cumin, coriander, paprika, and garlic for 3 minutes. Add the red wine vinegar and olive oil and mix for 1 minute. Season the mixture with salt to taste.
½ teaspoon coriander	
1 teaspoon paprika	
4 cloves garlic, minced	
2 tablespoons red wine vinegar	*3* Pour the mixture over the chicken pieces and coat. Marinate in the refrigerator for at least 30 minutes.
2 tablespoons olive oil	*4* Lightly grease the grill grates with oil and then heat the grill over medium-high heat. Skewer the chicken pieces and grill for 6 to 8 minutes on each side or until cooked thoroughly. Place on a serving dish and top with the cilantro.
Salt to taste	
½ cup cilantro, chopped	

Per serving: *Calories 262 (From fat 132); Total fat 15 g (Saturated 2 g); Protein 29 g; Carbohydrate 2 g (Dietary fiber 1 g); Cholesterol 87 mg; Sodium 155 mg.*

Tip: If you use wooden skewers, be sure to soak them in water ahead of time so they don't burn.

Source: Mediterranean Diet Cookbook For Dummies

Quick and Easy Dinners

Here are a few recipes that are quickly made even if you are late home from work. If you have the ingredients on hand, all but the Heart-Healthy Beef Stroganoff can be made in 30 minutes or less. A little simmering time is the only reason that the stroganoff takes 45 minutes.

Featuring fish

I love fish — both as a cardiologist and a food lover. Studies show substituting fish for red meat significantly lowers the amount of saturated fat in your diet and has a positive effect on lowering cholesterol levels and the risk of heart disease. This benefit is thought to be a result of the omega-3 fatty acids in fish combined with other nutrients also present in fish. The American Heart Association recommends that most people eat two servings (3.5 ounces per serving) of fish a week.

Fish with higher amounts of omega 3's include wild caught salmon, sardines, herring, tuna, and lake trout, although most fish have at least some.

Because there is concern about mercury in some fish, you should avoid eating fish that typically have higher levels of mercury, such as swordfish, king mackerel, tilefish, and shark. Each state publishes advisories about mercury in locally caught fish. The FDA and EPA recommend that pregnant women, breastfeeding mothers, and small children limit their intake of fish to avoid mercury. You can find more information about national fish safety advisories by going to http://www.epa.gov and entering "Fish Advisories" in the website's search box.

I also recommend eating fish responsibly from sustainable fisheries. You'll find good information about individual fish and types of fish at http://www.fishwatch.gov. Fish markets, both independent and in supermarkets, also provide information about where their fish and seafood come from. Never hesitate to ask questions, either.

Angel Hair Pasta with Fresh Tomatoes, Basil, and Garlic

Prep time: 10 min • **Cook time:** 15 min • **Yield:** 4 servings

Ingredients	Directions
4 ripe red tomatoes, blanched, peeled, seeded, and chopped	**1** Fill a large bowl with cold water and ice cubes. Set aside.
8 ounces angel hair pasta	
4 teaspoons extra virgin olive oil	**2** Fill a medium saucepan three-fourths with water and place on stove over high heat. Bring the water to a boil. Carefully drop the tomatoes into the boiling water and blanch for 30 seconds or until the skins start to crack. Using a slotted spoon, remove the tomatoes from the boiling water and place them in the ice water bath to stop the cooking process.
2 tablespoons fresh basil, destemmed and chopped	
2 cloves fresh garlic, minced	
Pepper to taste	
2 springs fresh basil, for garnish	**3** After you remove the tomatoes from the water, add the pasta. Cook until al dente, about 4 to 5 minutes or according to package instructions.
Freshly grated Parmesan cheese (optional)	
	4 Remove the tomatoes from the ice water after 1 minute and peel. Cut the tomatoes in half and squeeze out the seeds; chop the flesh of the tomatoes and set aside.
	5 When the pasta is cooked, drain and combine it with the tomatoes, olive oil, basil, and garlic in a large serving bowl. Toss together. Top with black pepper and garnish with basil. Top with freshly grated Parmesan cheese if desired. Serve immediately.

Per serving: Calories 294 (From fat 54); Total fat 6 g (Saturated 2 g); Protein 9 g; Carbohydrate 52 g (Dietary fiber 4 g); Cholesterol 0 mg; Sodium 13 mg.

Tip: This light dish is perfect for a hot summer night when served with a green salad and fresh fruit. Make a heartier dish by tossing in some warm roasted chicken or boiled shrimp (perhaps from leftovers) just before serving.

Vary It! Make the angel hair pasta whole grain. Whole wheat, buckwheat, or quinoa pastas are available in most supermarkets.

Source: Heart Healthy Cookbook For Dummies

Heart-Healthy Beef Stroganoff

Prep time: 20 min • **Cook time:** 25 min • **Yield:** 6 servings

Ingredients	*Directions*
1 tablespoon olive oil	*1* Bring a large pot of water to a boil and season with salt.
3 cloves garlic, minced	
1 small onion, chopped	*2* Heat the olive oil in a large skillet or sauté pan over medium-high heat. When the oil is hot, add the garlic and onion and sauté for 30 to 45 seconds, until aromatic, being careful not to let the garlic burn.
1 pound top round steak, trimmed of all visible fat and cut into 1 x ½ x ¼-inch slices	
1 tablespoon all-purpose flour	*3* In a medium bowl, toss the sliced beef with the flour, salt, and pepper. Add the seasoned beef to the pan, raise the heat to high, and cook for 3 to 5 minutes or until the beef is browned.
8 ounces mushrooms, sliced into ¼-inch slices	
½ cup red wine (any oak barrel aged red wine such as Merlot or Cabernet Sauvignon)	*4* Reduce the heat to medium-high and add the sliced mushrooms. Sauté, stirring often, for 2 to 3 minutes or until the mushrooms soften slightly.
½ cup low-fat sour cream	*5* Add the wine and cook for 1 minute to allow the alcohol to burn off; then add the sour cream, nutmeg, and thyme.
¼ teaspoon nutmeg, freshly ground, if possible	
¼ teaspoon thyme	*6* Reduce the heat to low and simmer for 10 minutes.
Salt and pepper to taste	
3 cups egg noodles	*7* While the beef simmers, drop the egg noodles in the boiling water and cook according to package directions. Drain and portion the noodles between six serving plates.
Fresh parsley, for garnish	
	8 To serve, spoon the beef mixture over the noodles and garnish with fresh parsley.

Per serving: Calories 373 (From fat 72); Total fat 8 g (Saturated 2 g); Protein 25 g; Carbohydrate 47 g (Dietary fiber 2.5 g); Cholesterol 99 mg; Sodium 64 mg.

Tip: If you need fewer than six servings for dinner, package extras in microwavable containers and take for lunch the next day.

Source: Healthy Heart Cookbook For Dummies

Moroccan Chicken with Tomatoes and Zucchini

Prep time: 5 min • **Cook time:** 25 min • **Yield:** 4 servings

Ingredients	Directions
Three 6-ounce boneless, skinless chicken breasts	*1* Cut the chicken breasts into bite-sized pieces (about 2 inches).
2 tablespoons olive oil	
6 cloves garlic, minced	*2* Heat a nonstick skillet over medium-high heat; add the olive oil, garlic, ginger, and chicken pieces, and cook for 5 minutes or until the chicken is browned on all sides.
1 teaspoon grated fresh ginger, or 1 teaspoon ground ginger	
2 zucchinis	*3* Meanwhile, cut the zucchinis lengthwise into quarters and chop into ½-inch moon shapes.
½ teaspoon pepper	
1 cup cilantro, chopped and divided	*4* Add the zucchini, ½ cup of the cilantro, and the canned tomatoes to the skillet; stir and cover for 15 minutes or until the chicken is cooked completely. Add the remaining cilantro and serve.
One 14.8-ounce can tomatoes, chopped	

Per serving: Calories 249 (From fat 95); Total fat 11 g (Saturated 2 g); Protein 30 g; Carbohydrate 9 g (Dietary fiber 2 g); Cholesterol 82 mg; Sodium 313 mg.

Tip: Try serving this dish over quick-cooking couscous or with curried rice.

Source: Mediterranean Diet Cookbook For Dummies

Sea Bass with Capers and Almond-Lemon Sauce

Prep time: 10 min • **Cook time:** 8 min • **Yield:** 4 servings

Ingredients	Directions
¼ cup breadcrumbs	*1* Pulse the breadcrumbs, almonds, garlic, lemon juice, and water in a food processor for 1 minute, scraping down the sides as needed. Gradually stream in the olive oil just until the sauce is creamy. Season with salt to taste. Set aside.
½ cup almonds	
2 cloves garlic	
¼ cup lemon juice	
¼ cup water	
¼ cup extra virgin olive oil	*2* Lightly season the sea bass with the salt. In a heavy skillet, heat olive oil and butter over medium heat. Add the capers and sea bass and cook for 4 minutes on each side. Remove the sea bass from the pan and place it on a serving platter; drizzle with the pan drippings.
Four 4- to 6-ounce sea bass fillets	
¼ teaspoon salt, plus more to taste	*3* Before serving, pour half the Almond-Lemon Sauce over the sea bass, leaving the remaining sauce to be added as desired.
1 tablespoon olive oil	
2 tablespoons butter	
2 tablespoons capers, drained and rinsed	

Per serving: Calories 431 (From fat 287); Total fat 32 g (Saturated 6 g); Protein 29 g; Carbohydrate 9 g (Dietary fiber 2 g); Cholesterol 60 mg; Sodium 435 mg.

Note: Although this recipe seems to contain a lot of fat, most of it comes from healthful olive oil and almonds. Eating both olive and nuts are associated with heart health.

Vary It! Although not included by the original author, I found the dish also tastes delicious if you don't make the original sauce, but start with Step 2 and then dress the cooked fish and capers with lemon juice and a little fresh, chopped parsley. You may also substitute any fish with firm, white flesh.

Source: Mediterranean Diet Cookbook For Dummies

Pasta Sauces for Quick Dinners

Most supermarkets offer a variety of whole grain pastas, ranging from whole wheat and buckwheat types to quinoa. You can fix dinner quickly by keeping on hand batches of the sauces I include in this section. Simply divide and freeze the sauces in portion sizes right for your family. Add a green salad to your pasta dish and serve fresh fruit for dessert for a simple, satisfying meal that tastes good and is good for you.

You can also use a smaller serving of pasta with pesto as a quick side dish with a roasted rotisserie chicken from the market.

Make it quick with pasta and leftovers

What do you do with one or two leftover cooked chicken breasts, a piece of grilled steak, a lone zucchini, two carrots, a couple of tomatoes (starting to wrinkle), and a stalk of broccoli in the vegetable drawer? The answer is simple — make a pasta dish for dinner. The leftovers will taste like a brand new dish! (To be ready, keep on hand two or three types of whole grain pasta that you like, extra virgin olive oil, toasted sesame oil, garlic, canned diced tomatoes (preferably low sodium), canned artichoke hearts or quarters, canned water chestnuts, dried or canned mushrooms, and capers. Keep the fridge stocked with lemons, green onions, and block Parmesan cheese.)

Here are some tasty main dishes you can make, selecting from these staples to fit the leftovers you have available. The approach for each type dish is flexible, so you don't need exact quantities — use your imagination and taste as you go:

✔ **Chicken salad:** Prepare bow-tie pasta. Slice or chunk leftover chicken into bite-sized pieces. Halve a handful of leftover grapes. Finely slice one green onion. Toss all the ingredients in a bowl with olive oil, lemon juice, Dijon mustard, and pepper to taste. Serve on lettuce leaves.

✔ **Steak salad:** Prepare spaghetti and toss with olive oil or toasted sesame oil and place in the fridge while you prepare the steak topping. Thinly slice leftover steak, quarter about 2 artichoke hearts per serving (remove any tough outer leaves), and finely slice one green onion per serving. Toss the steak and vegetables in a bowl with the lemon juice and olive or sesame oil (whichever you used on the pasta). Portion the spaghetti onto plates and serve the steak salad on top.

✔ **Pasta primavera:** Put the pasta on to cook. Then slice or dice your leftover vegetables such as carrots, yellow or zucchini squash, asparagus, tomatoes (large, cherry or drained canned), and broccoli flowerets. In a large nonstick skillet, sauté a sliced clove of garlic and add the sliced vegetables, starting with those that take longest to cook, such as carrots, and adding others as you go. Cook the vegetables until they are just tender. Add tomatoes at the very last. Toss the cooked vegetables and drained pasta with lemon juice, more olive oil if necessary, and salt and pepper. Top with grated or slivered Parmesan cheese.

Pesto Sauce

Prep time: 10 min • **Yield:** 8 servings

Ingredients	Directions
5 cups basil	*1* In a food processor, pulse the basil, garlic, and red chili pepper flakes ten times. Add the pine nuts and cheese and blend for 1 minute.
3 to 6 cloves garlic, crushed	
¼ teaspoon red pepper flakes	
½ cup pine nuts	*2* With the food processor on, slowly drizzle in the olive oil, adding more if needed. Season with salt and serve.
1 cup grated Parmesan cheese	
½ cup olive oil	
Salt to taste	

Per serving: Calories 235 (From fat 207); Total fat 23 g (Saturated 4 g); Protein 7 g; Carbohydrate 2 g (Dietary fiber 1 g); Cholesterol 11 mg; Sodium 192 mg.

Tip: You can keep pesto in the refrigerator for a week; be sure to store it with a top layer of olive oil. You can also freeze pesto for three months. (Olive oil on the surface is not needed when freezing.)

Tip: To preserve the bright green color of the basil in your pesto, drop the leaves in 4 quarts of boiling water for 20 seconds and then quickly strain them and place them in ice water. Drain and pat the leaves dry to remove excess water.

Vary It! Try these variations: Replace half the basil with arugula and the pine nuts with walnuts; replace the basil with cilantro, the pine nuts with almonds, and the Parmesan with manchego cheese; replace half the basil with spinach and the pine nuts with walnuts or almonds.

Source: Mediterranean Diet Cookbook For Dummies

Meat Sauce

Prep time: 10 min • **Cook time:** 46 min • **Yield:** 6 servings

Ingredients	Directions
1 tablespoon olive oil	**1** Heat the oil in a large, heavy skillet over medium-high heat. Add the ground beef and sprinkle with the salt. Cook the beef until brown, about 3 to 5 minutes, breaking it up with fork. Using a slotted spoon, transfer the beef to a plate.
1 pound lean ground beef	
½ teaspoon salt	
1 large onion, chopped	
3 cloves garlic, minced	**2** Add the onions and garlic to the skillet and sauté until the onion is tender, about 5 minutes. (Depending on how lean your beef is, you may need to add a teaspoon of oil to the pan.) Stir in the parsley, basil, and oregano and cook 1 minute.
1 teaspoon dried parsley, or 2 tablespoons fresh	
2 teaspoons dried basil, crumbled, or ¼ cup fresh	
2 teaspoons dried oregano, crumbled, or ¼ cup fresh	**3** Return the beef to the skillet and stir in the tomatoes, tomato sauce, and sugar. Reduce the heat to medium-low and simmer until the sauce is thick, about 45 minutes.
One 28-ounce can Italian diced tomatoes, drained	
One 8-ounce can tomato sauce	
1 teaspoon sugar	

Per serving: Calories 232 (From fat 125); Total fat 14 g (Saturated 5 g); Protein 16 g; Carbohydrate 12 g (Dietary fiber 2 g); Cholesterol 51 mg; Sodium 545 mg.

Tip: Sugar is often added to sauces to decrease the bitterness of the tomatoes. You can eliminate the sugar by adding ½ cup shredded carrots when you add the onion.

Vary It! Although this suggestion is not in the original recipe, you can also make this meat sauce with lean ground turkey or chicken. For a heartier flavor, add 1 teaspoon of soy sauce and 1 teaspoon of Worcestershire sauce to the turkey or chicken as you brown it.

Source: Mediterranean Diet Cookbook For Dummies

Chapter 19

Snacks, Starters, and Desserts

In This Chapter

▶ Making heart-healthy snacks and starters

▶ Discovering desserts that are both nutrient-rich and delicious

Here's good news! Snacks and desserts can play an important role in a heart-healthy diet. Unfortunately, most of the snacks and desserts available for purchase in the store tend to be energy dense without contributing much to good nutrition. Therefore, in this chapter, I provide some recipes that are both tasty and nutritious. That's even true of the recipe for brownies!

Also, note that all the recipes for snacks can be used as appetizers or starters before a meal. The same goes for the fruit soups that are part of the dessert section. Enjoy!

Snacks and Starters

The recipes in this section are easy-to-make and can serve as either a hearty, nutritious snack or an appetizer. Serve the dips and salsa with any of the following for a healthy snack:

✔ The Toasted Pita Chips (you can find the recipe in this chapter)

✔ Whole grain baked crackers or corn chips

✔ Fresh vegetable chunks (crudités), such as baby-cut carrots, celery sticks, broccoli and cauliflower flowerets, red and green pepper strips, yellow and zucchini slices, and jicama sticks

Spicy White Bean Dip

Prep time: 10 min • **Yield:** 8 servings (¼ cup each)

Ingredients	Directions
One 19-ounce can cannellini (white kidney) beans, rinsed and drained	*1* In the bowl of a food processor, combine beans, garlic, lemon juice, Tabasco sauce, and paprika; puree. Add water to thin the dip to the desired consistency.
2 cloves garlic	
1 teaspoon fresh lemon juice	*2* Transfer the dip to a serving dish, garnish with parsley, and serve with whole grain crackers.
2 to 3 drops Tabasco sauce (optional)	
¼ teaspoon paprika	
¼ cup water (optional)	
Sprig of parsley for garnish	
Whole grain crackers	

Per serving: Calories 74 (From fat 0); Total fat 0 g (Saturated 0 g); Protein 5 g; Carbohydrate 13 g (Dietary fiber 4 g); Cholesterol 0 mg; Sodium 137.

Tip: This dip also goes well with Toasted Pita Chips, which you can find later in this chapter.

Source: Healthy Heart Cookbook For Dummies

Star beans in starters

Beans are nutritional powerhouses. They are also wonderfully convenient because more than a dozen varieties are readily available canned. All you have to do is open, drain, rinse, and start creating a dip or salsa. For making dips, a food processor is handy. Here are some suggestions for quick bean-based starters:

✔ Substitute pinto beans or black beans in the Spicy White Bean Dip recipe. Add a handful of pitted black olives such as kalamatas to the black bean dip before processing. With pinto bean dip, stir in small chunks of avocado to the dip after it's finished.

✔ Make a spicy bean salsa. Choose any bean or combo of beans you like (drained and rinsed), add a can of tomatoes with chiles (include some or all of the liquid), a can of drained kernel corn, and a tablespoon or two of chopped cilantro. Other variants include diced red and green peppers, diced sweet onion, and/or small avocado chunks.

Green Pimento and Mango Salsa

Prep time: 25 min • **Yield:** 8 servings (⅓ cup)

Ingredients	Directions
2 green bell peppers	**1** Halve and seed the green peppers. Arrange the pepper halves on a baking sheet, skin side up, and place under broiler for 3 to 4 minutes until the skin blisters and blackens; rotate the pan if necessary for even cooking.
1½ cup ripe, fresh mango, peeled and diced	
½ cup red bell pepper, diced	
¼ to ½ cup diced hot pickled cherry peppers (Italian style in vinegar, not oil)	**2** Place the roasted peppers into a bag and close it (or into a bowl and cover tightly with plastic wrap). Set aside for 10 minutes to loosen the skins.
½ cup pineapple juice	
2 tablespoons red wine vinegar	**3** Peel the pepper halves, discard the skins, and dice. Use ½ cup for this recipe.
2 tablespoons fresh cilantro, chopped	
2 tablespoons fresh basil, chopped	**4** Combine all ingredients in a glass bowl and let sit for at least 30 minutes.
Salt to taste (analysis based on ¼ teaspoon)	
Freshly ground black pepper to taste	

Per serving: Calories 50 (From fat 0); Total fat 0 g (Saturated 0 g); Protein 0 g; Carbohydrate 12 g (Dietary fiber 2 g); Cholesterol 0 mg; Sodium 274 mg.

Tip: Serve this salsa with baked tortilla chips or Toasted Pita Chips (you can find the recipe in this chapter). It also makes a good sauce for broiled or grilled chicken or fish.

Tip: If you have more than ½ cup roasted, diced pepper, freeze it to toss into Spicy Pinto Bean Chili (Chapter 17) or the Meat Sauce (Chapter 18) for pasta.

Source: Heart Disease For Dummies

Hummus

Prep time: 10 min • **Yield:** 16 servings

Ingredients	*Directions*
Two 14.5-ounce cans chickpeas	*1* Drain the chickpeas and reserve ¼ to ½ cup of the liquid. Place the chickpeas in a food processor and puree until smooth.
Juice of 2 lemons	
2 cloves garlic	*2* Add the remaining ingredients and blend until the mixture is creamy. If necessary, add the liquid reserved from the canned chickpeas to create the desired creaminess. Transfer the hummus to a bowl and serve.
¼ tablespoon olive oil	
¼ cup tahini paste	
½ teaspoon salt	
Pinch of cayenne pepper	

Per serving: Calories 85 (From fat 25); Total fat 3g (Saturated 0 g); Protein 3 g; Carbohydrate 12 g (Dietary fiber 2 g); Cholesterol 0 mg; Sodium 228 mg.

Tip: Serve with Toasted Pita Chips (see the recipe in this chapter) or fresh vegetables such as carrots.

Note: Store hummus in a glass container in the refrigerator for up to a week. Cover the surface of the hummus with a thin layer of olive oil.

Note: Tahini paste is made from ground sesame seeds. It is a major component of hummus and other Middle Eastern dishes. You can find tahini paste at most grocery stores or specialty stores near the cooking oils or possibly in the stores' ethnic sections. If you can't find it in your store, look for it online at Amazon.com.

Source: Mediterranean Diet Cookbook For Dummies

Baba Gannoujh (Roasted Eggplant Dip)

Prep time: 5 min • **Cook time:** 30 min • **Yield:** 16 servings

Ingredients	Directions
2 large eggplants	**1** Preheat the oven to 450 degrees. Line a baking sheet with foil.
½ cup tahini paste	
2 cloves garlic	**2** Poke the eggplant once with a fork on all sides to allow the steam to escape during cooking. Bake the eggplant on a baking sheet for about 30 minutes or until soft. Remove the eggplant from the oven and cool until you can comfortably touch it.
Juice of 2 lemons	
3 tablespoons water	
1 tablespoon extra virgin olive oil	
1 teaspoon salt	**3** Cut the eggplant in half. Scoop out the inside of the eggplant with a spoon, discarding the skin.
2 tablespoons fresh parsley, chopped, for serving	
	4 Pulse the cooked eggplant in a food processor for 1 minute. Add the tahini, garlic, lemon juice, water, olive oil, and salt to the eggplant mixture and blend until you achieve a thicker consistency. Transfer to a serving bowl, garnish with the chopped parsley, and serve with pita chips.

Per serving: Calories 68 (From fat 45); Total fat 5 g (Saturated 1 g); Protein 2 g; Carbohydrate 6 g (Dietary fiber 3 g); Cholesterol 0 mg; Sodium 149 mg.

Source: Mediterranean Diet Cookbook For Dummies

Toasted Pita Chips

Prep time: 5 min • **Cook time:** 12–15 minutes • **Yield:** 4 servings

Ingredients	Directions
4 whole wheat pitas	*1* Preheat the oven to 375 degrees.
4 teaspoons olive oil	
Sea salt to taste	*2* Using a pastry brush, brush each pita with 1 teaspoon of olive oil. Sprinkle with sea salt to taste.
	3 Cut each pita into 8 wedges. Arrange the pita wedges on a baking sheet and bake for 12 to 15 minutes. Cool the pita chips to room temperature and serve.

Per serving: Calories 210 (From fat 55); Total fat 6 g (Saturated 1 g); Protein 6 g; Carbohydrate 35 g (Dietary fiber 5 g); Cholesterol 0 mg; Sodium 341.

Source: Mediterranean Diet Cookbook For Dummies

More healthy dippers and snacks

Toasted whole wheat pita chips make great dippers for salsas, hummus, and other low-fat dips. Here are other healthful options for dippers or snacks:

✔ **Whole grain crackers and bruschetta made from whole-grain baguettes:** These are great for dips but also good spread with a nut butter.

✔ **Unusual vegetable dippers:** Jicama slices, sliced water chestnuts, fresh artichoke leaves all make good options. Cook a fresh artichoke and let guests pull leaves to dip.

✔ **The usual vegetable suspects:** Carrots sliced diagonally, celery sticks, green and red pepper strips, sliced radishes, sliced summer squash, broccoli and cauliflower flowerets — these are familiar but tasty with dips or salsas or by themselves.

✔ **Air-popped popcorn or low-fat microwave popcorn.** Popcorn is a great whole grain snack anytime. If you air pop, use butter flakes rather than the real thing.

✔ **A handful of nuts.** A handful — about ¼ cup — is packed with nutrients.

✔ **Your own trail mix.** Combine a whole grain cereal (such as oat circles or whole wheat squares), raisins and dried blueberries, and a selection of nuts (pecans, peanuts, walnuts, almonds, and pistachios are good).

Desserts

The right dessert can make a good meal seem even more special. The recipes in this section offer treats that are sweet but, when compared to most desserts, are low in calories and provide many nutrients. As you may have guessed, fruit plays a major role in each recipe. Three take only a few minutes to make and the other two a bit more time. All are worth the effort.

Recently, I saw a T-shirt with the slogan "Life is Short. Eat dessert first!" We laugh, but the phrase also points out something that should be true of healthful eating plans: They must be pleasurable as well as healthful. That's the beauty of desserts like those I share here. Taking these desserts as models, you might review some of your favorite dessert recipes to see which are similar and which you might modify. Also remember that from time to time there's room for the most indulgent dessert in your repertoire.

Going for chocolate

Dark chocolate can be good for you. Research has confirmed that dark chocolate is a rich source of antioxidant flavonoids. The nonfat cocoa solids provide these antioxidants, not the cocoa butter (fat). So enjoying a little square of dark chocolate as a quick dessert can be good for you. Chocolate with higher percentages of cocoa, like bittersweet, typically has less sugar.

Eating a little bit of dark chocolate daily has been associated with decreased LDL cholesterol, reduced risk of heart attack, decreased blood pressure, and increased insulin sensitivity. Does this mean you should pig out on dark chocolate every day? No, but it does mean that you can enjoy it regularly in a balanced nutrition plan. Just watch out for chocolate foods with lots of added sugar and noncocoa fats.

Homemade chocolate meringues are one guilt-free treat I like to make. Here's the basic technique that you can use to adapt a recipe you like. It has no added fat or sugar. Whip the whites of 4 eggs to a stiff peak. Add to taste a noncaloric sweetener (½ to 1 packet) — either sucralose or stevia work best because they don't break down with heat. Fold in 1 to 2 tablespoons of cocoa powder. The more cocoa powder, the stronger the chocolate flavor. Drop by teaspoonful on a greased cookie sheet and bake in a low to medium oven (250–300 degrees) for 30 to 35 minutes. Meringues should be light and crunchy, not sticky or chewy, after cooling on a rack. Store in an airtight container for a week or so (they won't last that long).

Dark Fudge Brownies

Prep time: 45 min • **Cook time:** 40 min • **Yield:** 24 servings

Ingredients	Directions
One 15-ounce can black beans, unseasoned, rinsed well and drained	**1** Preheat the oven to 350 degrees. Coat a 9-x-13-inch baking pan with cooking spray.
1 cup pureed prunes (or prune filling or prune-based oil substitute)	**2** Blend the drained beans and pureed prunes in a food processor until very smooth. Add the egg whites, blend again, and set aside. If you don't have a food processor, use a blender to blends the beans, prunes, and egg whites until very smooth.
6 egg whites	
¾ cup unsweetened cocoa powder	**3** Melt the margarine in a small saucepan on the stove or in the microwave. Stir in the cocoa and canola oil until well blended.
3 tablespoons canola oil	
1 tablespoon stick margarine, trans fat free	**4** Combine the bean mixture, sugar, flour, and egg whites in a mixing bowl and stir until well combined. Add the cocoa mixture and stir again.
1½ cups granulated sugar	
¼ cup all-purpose flour	**5** Pour the mixture into the baking pan and sprinkle the top with walnuts.
1 teaspoon pure vanilla extract	
½ cup walnuts, chopped	**6** Bake for 35 to 40 minutes. Cook completely before cutting into 24 squares.
Nonstick cooking spray	
	7 Store the brownies in an airtight container in the refrigerator for up to 1 week.

Per serving: Calories 137 (From fat 36); Total fat 4 g (Saturated 0.5 g); Protein 4 g; Carbohydrate 24 g (Dietary fiber 3 g); Cholesterol 0 mg; Sodium 21 mg.

Note: The secret to these rich and decadent yet low-fat brownies is the black beans. Wait, wait, wait! Before you flip the page, give these brownies a chance. You'll be surprised and delighted by the rich chocolate flavor and fudge-like texture of these good-for-you treats.

Source: Healthy Heart Cookbook For Dummies

Phyllo-Crusted Berry Cobbler

Prep time: 15 min • **Cook time:** 30 min, plus 15 min to cool • **Yield:** 4 servings

Ingredients	Directions
2 pints berries (blackberries, raspberries, and blueberries)	*1* Preheat the oven to 350 degrees.
2 packets artificial sweetener (see note)	*2* Toss the berries with the artificial sweetener, flour, and lemon juice. Place in an adequately sized ovenproof dish (about 6-x-9 inches).
1 tablespoon all purpose flour	
1 tablespoon lemon juice	
1 tablespoon apple juice concentrate	*3* Brush phyllo dough with melted margarine and sprinkle with granulated sugar. Layer all 4 sheets of phyllo in this manner. Loosely crumple the phyllo and place on top of the berry mixture.
4 sheets phyllo dough	
1 tablespoon light margarine, melted	*4* Bake until golden brown and berries begin to bubble, about 30 minutes.
1 tablespoon granulated sugar	*5* Allow to cool for 15 minutes and then serve.

Per serving: Calories 225 (From fat 27); Total fat 3 g (Saturated 1 g); Protein 3 g; Carbohydrate 50 g (Dietary fiber 10 g); Cholesterol 0 mg; Sodium 117 mg.

Note: Some artificial sweeteners, especially ones made with aspartame, break down when exposed to high heat. A recipe like this one is best made with a heat-stable artificial sweetener such as sucralose or stevia.

Source: Healthy Heart Cookbook For Dummies

Chilled Strawberry Soup with Champagne

Prep time: 20 min, plus 4 hrs chilling time • **Cook time:** 1 min • **Yield:** 4 servings

Ingredients	Directions
4 ounces (9 tablespoons) sugar	**1** Boil the water with the sugar for 1 minute to create a simple syrup. Set the syrup aside to cool.
½ cup water	
2 pints strawberries	**2** Wash the strawberries and cut off the stems. Cut 4 of the strawberries into quarters and set aside for garnish. Place the remaining strawberries in a blender with the simple syrup and blend well to get a smooth consistency.
8 mint leaves	
4 mint sprigs for garnish	
1 cup Champagne (or sparkling cider)	**3** Cut mint leaves into thin strips (julienne).
2 tablespoons powdered sugar	**4** Pour the strawberry soup into a bowl, add the mint strips, and refrigerate for 4 hours, until the soup is very cold and the flavors are blended.
	5 When the soup is ready to serve, pour in the Champagne and mix well.
	6 Ladle the soup into chilled individual serving bowls.
	7 In each bowl, arrange four strawberry quarters to form a star and garnish with a mint spring in the center of the star.
	8 Dust with powdered sugar and serve.

Per serving: Calories 208 (From fat 4); Total fat 0.5 g (Saturated 0); Protein 1 g; Carbohydrate 43 g (Dietary fiber 3 g); Cholesterol 0 mg; Sodium 7 mg.

Tip: When you want an elegant but light finish to a meal, try this strawberry soup. It is very easy to make but the presentation will wow family or friends.

Source: Healthy Heart Cookbook For Dummies

Red Fruits Soup

Prep time: 10 min • **Cook time:** 5 min • **Yield:** 4 servings

Ingredients	Directions
1½ cups red wine	*1* Place the wine, lemon juice, and sugar in a stainless-steel (noncorrosive) saucepan and bring to a boil.
Juice from 1 lemon	
2 tablespoons sugar	*2* Add the fruits and bring to a low boil.
6 ounces (1¼ cup) frozen sour cherries, thawed	*3* In a small bowl, combine the water and arrowroot; heat well in a saucepan until the arrowroot is dissolved. Pour this mixture over the fruit, stir, and cook for 1 minute longer.
6 ounces (1¼ cup) raspberries, fresh or frozen, thawed	
6 ounces (1¼ cup) strawberries, fresh	
3 tablespoons cold water	*4* Remove the soup from the heat and chill before serving.
1 teaspoon arrowroot	

Per serving: Calories 144 (From fat 0); Total fat 0 g (Saturated 0 g); Protein 1 g; Carbohydrate 22 g (Dietary fiber 4 g); Cholesterol 0 mg; Sodium 6 mg.

Source: Healthy Heart Cookbook For Dummies

In a hurry? Go for ambrosia

One of the simplest desserts — also delicious and nutritious — is ambrosia. If you think ambrosia requires whipped toppings and marshmallows, stop right there and think again. The most heavenly combo is nothing more than a chilled mixture of segmented oranges with their juice and fresh grated coconut (although unsweetened packaged grated coconuts works fine). The flavors meld wonderfully if you make it the day before and let it chill overnight, but right before the guests arrive is also fine. If you want to give it a try, aim for one orange per serving and about a tablespoon of grated or flaked coconut.

Flexibility is another great thing about ambrosia. You can vary the mixture with other fresh fruits. Here are some mixtures I enjoy:

- Orange segments, small pineapple chunks, and grated coconut.

- Orange segments, apple bits (slice the apple, then dice the slice), chopped pecans, and grated coconut

- Orange and grapefruit segments, pitted fresh cherries (halved), and grated coconut.

Poached Pears with Orange Yogurt Sauce

Prep time: 30 min • **Cook time:** About 25 min • **Yield:** 6 servings

Ingredients	*Directions*
4 cups orange Muscat wine 2 cups blossom honey	*1* In a large saucepan, combine the wine, honey, cinnamon, and cardamom and simmer for 10 minutes.
1 cinnamon stick 10 cardamom seeds	*2* Add the pears and poach until they are tender, about 12 minutes.
6 ripe pears peeled, halved, and cored Orange Yogurt Sauce (see the following recipe)	*3* Place the pan in an ice bath to cool the pears and poaching liquid. While the pears cool, prepare the Orange Yogurt Sauce.
½ cup chopped pistachios, for garnish	*4* Line six plates with the yogurt sauce (see the following recipe).
6 sprigs of mint, for garnish	*5* Drain the poached pears on paper towels and then place 2 pear halves on each plate.
	6 Garnish with chopped pistachios and mint.

Orange Yogurt Sauce

1 cup low-fat vanilla yogurt	*1* Grate the zest off the orange and then juice the orange.
1 orange 2 tablespoons Grand Marnier liqueur	*2* Whisk together the yogurt, orange juice, zest, and Grand Marnier. Set aside until ready to use.

Per serving: Calories 284 (From fat 54); Total fat 6 g (Saturated 1 g); Protein 5 g; Carbohydrate 51 g (Dietary fiber 6 g); Cholesterol 2 mg; Sodium 110 mg.

Tip: Cardamom is a tropical spice related to ginger and has a spicy-sweet flavor. It is used widely in Indian and Scandinavian cooking. Although it comes ground, get the seed if you can because the ground spice loses flavor quickly.

Source: Healthy Heart Cookbook For Dummies

Part VI
The Part of Tens

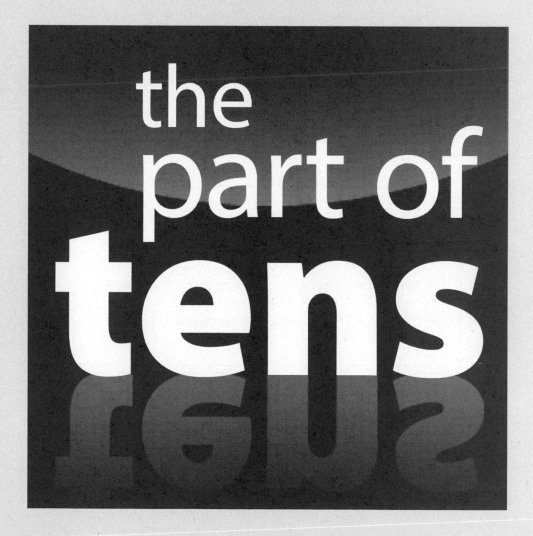

For a bonus Part of Tens chapter on how to prevent and reverse heart disease, head to www.dummies.com/extras/preventingreversingheartdisease.

In this part . . .

- Find out how women may experience heart disease differently than men.

- Check out cardiac symptoms and signs you should know about and never ignore.

- Review common tests used in evaluating heart disease and consider when they are useful and when they aren't.

- Discover ways to help involve family members of all ages in a heart-healthy lifestyle.

Chapter 20

Ten Differences in Heart Disease between Women and Men

. . . .

In This Chapter

▶ Understanding how risk factors may differ in women

▶ Exploring different manifestations of heart disease

. . . .

For many years the majority of women and their doctors underestimated the risk of heart disease. Few understood that heart disease was the number one cause of death for women, as it is for men. Thanks to public health campaigns, women are growing more aware. By 2012, 56 percent of women identified heart disease as the leading cause of death for their gender. That's up from only 36 percent in 1997, only 15 years previously. However, this knowledge is still very low in some groups: only 36 percent of African-American women and 34 percent of Hispanic women identified heart disease as the leading cause of death in women.

The information in this book can help women as well as men learn how to prevent heart disease and reverse risk factors for it. When it comes to heart disease and its risk factors, men and women have much in common. But there are also some important differences. If you are a woman, understanding these differences can help you partner with your doctor to do the best you can to prevent or beat heart disease.

Women Tend to Develop CHD Later than Men

On average, women develop heart disease ten years later than men. Until about age 55, women overall have a lower risk and incidence of diagnosed coronary heart disease than men. Before menopause, natural levels of estrogen appear to play a role in slowing down the manifestations of heart disease. After menopause, however, women's risk increases significantly until it is equal to or greater than that in men.

Research has shown more recently that hormone replacement therapy does not lower the risk of CHD and may actually pose health risks.

Although the manifestations of heart disease may arrive later in women, you must remember that heart disease is still the number 1 cause of death for women just as it is for men. Also, women have the same primary risk factors as men, and these often begin in early life, even in childhood. At least 75 percent of women ages 40 to 60 have at least one major risk factor for heart disease. Some of these risk factors, such as diabetes and smoking, also pose greater CHD risks in women than men. Fortunately, adopting lifestyle measures to reduce risk factors dramatically slows the development of heart disease and lowers your risk of a heart attack or stroke.

Women May Experience Different Warning Signs

Many women who have coronary heart disease, like most men, may experience angina as chest pain or discomfort that occurs with activity and stops when activity ceases. However, many women may have more diffuse or subtle signs of angina, such as the following:

- Discomfort or pain that appears in the neck, jaw, or upper back
- Feeling very short of breath
- Nausea, vomiting, or abdominal distress that may feel like indigestion or acid reflux.

Such symptoms may occur with or without chest discomfort. More women may also experience these temporary symptoms when they are asleep or resting, not just during activity. If you experience any of these symptoms, immediately have your doctor evaluate you for heart disease.

The most common warning sign of heart attack for many women, like men, is a feeling of tightness, pressure, or pain in the center of the chest that lasts longer than a few minutes. But many women also have more diffuse or subtle warning symptoms. These include fatigue; pain in the jaw, neck, upper back, abdomen, or one or both; shortness of breath; experiencing nausea or vomiting; breaking out in a cold sweat; or experiencing lightheadedness or dizziness. Women experiencing such symptoms may ignore them because they don't resemble the classic sign of chest pain or because they don't seem very severe. However, if you experience any of these symptoms for more than five minutes, treat the situation as an emergency — call 911. Don't drive yourself or allow a family member to drive you to the hospital.

Many Women Experience CHD as Microvascular Disease

Up to 50 percent of women with cardiac symptoms who have a heart catheterization screening have no blockages in the major arteries of the heart. Instead, their symptoms arise from *coronary microvascular disease (MVD)*. In MVD the tiny arteries of the heart, those about the diameter of a human hair or slightly larger, are damaged in ways that restrict the flow of blood to the heart muscle.

Having high blood pressure before menopause, particularly systolic high blood pressure (the upper number), increases a woman's risk of having MVD. Unfortunately, the standard tests for coronary heart disease, ranging from stress testing to heart catheterization, aren't designed to measure blood flow in these very small vessels. That's one reason that it has taken the medical profession a relatively long time to understand how common MVD is in women and to increase research to better diagnose and treat it. It's very clear, however, that the same risk factors that contribute to atherosclerosis in the larger arteries also contribute to microvascular disease. So controlling these risk factors is also a first line strategy to prevent MVD in the first place and to manage the condition if you have it.

Diabetes May Increase the Risk of CHD More in Women

Almost 9 percent of American women age 20 or older have type 2 diabetes (4.7 percent of white women, 12.6 percent of African American women, and 11.3 percent of Mexican American women). Particularly in women younger than age 60, having diabetes has been associated with a greater risk of having cardiovascular disease than for men with diabetes.

Having diabetes seems to remove the approximately 10-year age advantage for the onset of heart disease that women in general experience over men (refer to the earlier section "Women Tend to Develop CHD Later than Men"). A recent meta-analysis also found that women with diabetes had a 44 percent greater chance of dying from a heart attack or stroke than did men with diabetes. The reasons for these observed differences are not clear. One suggested contributing factor is that many women may be less likely than men to have diagnoses of other CHD risk factors and thus have less control of them. Research has begun into other potential differences in men and women with diabetes, such as any biological gender differences.

Women May Experience More Problems with Statin Medications

Statin medications can significantly lower elevated LDL cholesterol and total cholesterol. Many studies show that taking statins has been associated with reduced risks of heart attack and mortality from heart disease in individuals who have risk factors. However, women have been very much underrepresented in clinical trials of statins. And there is conflicting evidence and continuing controversy that taking statins to lower LDL benefits healthy women without manifestations of CHD.

Yet, a higher percentage of women than men experience serious side effects from taking statins, particularly larger doses. Such side effects include muscle and joint pain, muscle weakness, and fatigue. Women taking statins have a greater risk than men of experiencing increased blood sugar and developing type 2 diabetes. Before starting statins for either primary or secondary prevention of CHD, thoroughly discuss with your doctor the potential benefits and drawbacks of statins for your individual circumstances.

Smoking Is a Greater Risk Factor for Heart Disease in Women

Women who smoke have a 25 percent greater risk of developing heart disease than men who smoke. In addition, middle-aged women smokers are more likely to have a heart attack than men smokers. How much more? About twice as likely. And the increased danger doesn't stop there. Women who smoke and take birth control pills may increase their risk even more. Smoking may also decrease HDL cholesterol (the good cholesterol) more in women than men.

But there's good news. If you quit smoking, you can reduce your risk of heart disease by half in just a year. The longer you stay quit, the better the picture.

Depression May Be a Greater CHD Risk Factor for Women

Population studies indicate that having depression is associated with a 50 to 100 percent greater risk of having heart disease. And women are about twice as likely to have depression as men. The reasons for the apparent link between depression and CHD are not yet clear, but depression can lead to negative ways of coping, such as eating poorly, smoking, and not being active — all of which increase your risk of developing CHD.

As a group, women are less likely to be physically active than men, whether they have depression or not. One recent study found the association between depression and heart disease was particularly prevalent in women aged 55 and under. This group of women also tend to have poorer outcomes after a heart attack. The possibility that depression may increase your risk of heart problems is another reason to seek help for this problem and not tough it out.

Gestational Diabetes and Hypertension Increase Risk of Later Developing CHD

Gestational diabetes and hypertension are temporary conditions that may occur during pregnancy for some women. Gestational diabetes occurs in an estimated 9 percent of pregnancies and gestational high blood pressure in an estimated 6 percent. In long-term observational studies, having either of these conditions has been associated with a greater risk that you will develop heart disease later in life. One recent study, for example, found early signs of cardiovascular disease in middle-aged women who had not developed diabetes but had experienced gestational diabetes. There is some evidence that gestational diabetes and hypertension also increase the risk of heart disease for the children born of the pregnancies. So what should you do? The most important thing is to get good prenatal care. Your obstetrician will check for these conditions and will work with you to control them should they occur.

Exercise Stress Tests May Not Be as Accurate in Women

Exercise stress testing using a treadmill or stationary cycle is a screening tool commonly used for diagnosing or ruling out heart disease for people who may be at risk of CHD or who have reported potential symptoms. Studies suggest that the results may often be misleading in women. One study, for example, found that results were not accurate in about 35 percent of women tested.

Results appear to be more accurate with nuclear exercise stress tests, in which a radioactive dye and nuclear images are taken before and after the exercise session. Some studies suggest that using either type of stress test with echocardiography may be the most accurate approach for many women. If you need screening, discuss these issues with your doctor.

Women Are More Likely to Die in the First Year after a Heart Attack

For reasons that aren't yet clear, more women than men tend to die in the first year after a heart attack. In succeeding years, the numbers are about equal. A number of factors may play a role in this unfortunate situation, including these two:

✔ Women sometimes delay getting treatment because they think they couldn't be having a heart attack.

✔ Women may be sicker when they have a heart attack. Some studies suggest that women may be less aggressively treated — diagnosed at a later age with heart disease, not treated as aggressively in the emergency department or with medicines, angioplasty or surgery, and not referred as often to rehabilitation.

Recently, significant efforts have been made to address such possible deficiencies, and although there has been improvement, women still lag men in recovery and response to interventions. Recent studies suggest this is especially true in women age 55 and under. These potential outcomes are another important reason to do all you can to prevent heart disease in the first place.

Chapter 21

Ten Cardiac Symptoms You Shouldn't Ignore

In This Chapter
▶ Understanding which symptoms suggest heart disease
▶ Knowing when to take symptoms to the doctor

Although medical signs and symptoms can overlap, you can distinguish between the two on the basis of who is experiencing them. For example, you may regard a nagging, worrisome cough as a *symptom*. Your doctor, however, may regard that cough as a *sign* of congestion of the lungs. In broad terms, then, *symptoms* are feelings or conditions that a patient experiences and then tries to describe to his or her physician. *Signs* are findings that the physician derives from the physical examination that point toward the proper cardiac diagnosis.

Depending on the circumstances and severity, some symptoms (conditions you experience) may represent signs of serious cardiac disease to your physician or may not be worrisome at all. In this chapter, I look at ten key symptoms and signs.

Chest Pain

Chest pain probably is the most common symptom for which people go to see a cardiologist. Although chest pain can signify heart problems, it also can stem from a wide variety of structures in the chest, neck, and back that have no relation (other than proximity) to the heart. The lungs, skin, muscles, spine, and portions of the gastrointestinal tract, such as the stomach, small bowel, pancreas, and gallbladder are among these structures. Pain caused by angina or heart attack usually is located beneath the breastbone but may also be located in the front of the chest or either arm, neck, cheeks, teeth, or high in the middle of the back. Exercise, strong emotion, or stress may also provoke chest pain. Very short bouts of pain lasting five to ten seconds typically are not angina or heart-related but are more likely to be musculoskeletal pain. If you have concern about *any* chest discomfort, going to a medical facility and having it further evaluated is imperative. (See Chapter 2 for more.)

Shortness of Breath

Shortness of breath is a major cardiac symptom. But determining whether this symptom comes from problems with the heart, the lungs, or some other organ system typically is difficult. Exertion can cause temporary shortness of breath in otherwise healthy individuals who are working or exercising strenuously or in sedentary individuals who are working even moderately. But an abnormally uncomfortable awareness of breathing or difficulty breathing can be a symptom of a medical problem. Shortness of breath that occurs when you're at rest, for example, is considered a strong cardiac symptom. If shortness of breath lasts longer than five minutes after activity or occurs when you're at rest, have your doctor evaluate it.

Loss of Consciousness

Loss of consciousness usually results from reduced blood supply to the brain. Perhaps the most common loss of consciousness is what people usually call a *fainting episode.* This temporary condition may be brought on by being in a warm or constricted environment or in a highly emotional state. Such episodes often are preceded by dizziness and/or a sense of *fading to black.* The condition may also be accompanied by nausea and a cold sweat.

When the heart is the cause, loss of consciousness typically occurs rapidly and without preceding events. Cardiac conditions ranging from rhythm disturbances (electrical problems in the heart) to mechanical problems potentially can cause fainting or a blackout. Because such cardiac problems can be serious, never dismiss the loss of consciousness in an otherwise healthy individual as a fainting episode until that person has a complete medical workup.

Cardiovascular Collapse

You can't experience a more dramatic symptom or greater emergency than *cardiovascular collapse,* also called *sudden cardiac death.* Of course, cardiovascular collapse results in a sudden loss of consciousness, but the victim typically has no pulse and stops breathing. The victim of a seizure or fainting spell, on the other hand, has a pulse and continues breathing. Cardiovascular collapse can occur as a complication in an individual who has known heart disease but sometimes may be the first manifestation of an acute heart attack or rhythm problem. When cardiovascular collapse occurs, resuscitation must take place within a very few minutes or death inevitably follows. Being able to respond quickly to cardiovascular collapse is the greatest reason for learning CPR or basic cardiac life support. Automated emergency defibrillators (AEDs) are increasingly available in public places; they are designed so that laypersons can use them, without training, to help save a life.

Palpitations

Palpitations, which can be defined as an unpleasant awareness of a rapid or forceful beating of the heart, may indicate anything from serious cardiac rhythm problems to nothing worrisome at all. Typically, an individual who is experiencing palpitations describes a sensation of a *skipped beat;* however, people also may describe a rapid heartbeat or a sensation of lightheadedness. Whenever the palpitation is accompanied by lightheadedness or loss of consciousness, a further workup is imperative to determine whether serious, underlying heart-rhythm problems are present. Often, the simplest underlying causes of palpitations can be turned around by getting more sleep, drinking less coffee or other caffeinated beverages, decreasing alcohol consumption, or trying to reduce the amount of stress in your life. Nevertheless, you need to take this problem to your doctor for evaluation first.

Edema

Edema is an abnormal accumulation of fluid in the body, a type of swelling, and has many causes. The location and distribution of the swelling is helpful for determining what causes it. If edema occurs in the legs, it usually is characteristic of heart failure or of problems with the veins of the legs. Edema with a cardiac origin typically is *symmetric,* which means that it involves both legs. An abnormal gathering of fluid in the lungs is called *pulmonary edema,* and the typical symptom is shortness of breath. This symptom also can be typical in a patient with heart failure. Abnormal gathering of fluid in either the legs or the lungs always indicates the need for a complete cardiac workup.

Cyanosis

Cyanosis, the bluish discoloration of the skin resulting from inadequate oxygen in the blood, is a sign and a symptom. One form of cyanosis occurs when unoxygenated blood that normally is pumped through the right side of the heart somehow passes into the left ventricle and is pumped out to the body. This anomaly commonly occurs in congenital abnormalities that create abnormal openings between the right and left sides of the heart. The second type of cyanosis commonly is caused by constriction of blood vessels in your limbs or peripheries and may be the result of a low output from the heart or from exposure to cold air or water. Whether the cyanosis is central or peripheral in nature guides a physician in the search for which type of underlying condition is causing the cyanosis. Any form of cyanosis is a symptom that should prompt discussion with your physician.

Cough

As anyone who has had a head cold knows, a cough can accompany a viral illness. It can also represent a variety of underlying causes such as cancers, allergies, abnormalities of the lungs, or abnormalities of the breathing tube. The cardiovascular disorders that result in cough are those that cause abnormal accumulations of fluid in the lungs, such as significant heart failure. Take any prolonged or unexplained cough to your doctor.

Coughing Up Blood

Coughing up blood of any kind — from small streaks in sputum to large quantities — is called *hemoptysis* in medicine. This condition can result from a variety of very serious diseases of the lungs or even some forms of cancer. Whatever the cause, coughing up blood-tinged secretions never is normal and may represent a medical emergency. If you ever cough up blood in any form, no matter how minor it seems, contact your doctor immediately.

Fatigue

In busy, hectic lives, *fatigue* may stem from a bewilderingly large number of underlying causes ranging from depression to side effects of drugs to physical illnesses, including cardiac problems. The ordinary fatigue you feel after working hard is normal, even when you have to crash into bed early. But a significant level of *enduring* fatigue should always prompt a call to your doctor, who may want to do an appropriate medical workup to determine possible underlying causes.

Chapter 22

Ten Heart Tests to Consider or Avoid

....

In This Chapter

▶ Profiling common tests to diagnose cardiac risk and conditions

▶ Understanding guidelines for when and for whom specific tests are appropriate

....

Diagnostic tests exist for almost all cardiac risk factors and heart conditions — often in what seems a bewildering variety. What's the primary purpose of such tests? In the broadest sense, these tests are designed to help healthcare professionals get a better understanding of heart conditions and heart health in individuals who may be experiencing symptoms of possible heart problems or to evaluate individuals who have such high risk of heart problems that further testing is warranted.

Because you have a vested interest in your heart health, you should certainly understand what some of the most common cardiac tests are. Because you want to partner with your doctors in getting the best care for your individual needs, you also should consider what tests may or may not be appropriate in various circumstances.

At present, debate continues among the medical and public health community about whether some types of tests are overused. Making the right decision often requires doctor and patient to balance between prevention and the dangers of false positives or even physical risks for healthy people without symptoms. Knowing more about the ten test procedures I cover in this chapter will prepare you to work with your doctors to make the choices that are right for you.

Blood Tests to Determine CHD Risk

In a regular checkup or follow-up visit, your physician typically orders a variety of basic blood analyses that are performed using one or two vials of blood drawn after you've been fasting for 8 to 12 hours. These tests are inexpensive and provide very good evaluation insights for your doctors. Tests that directly relate to the heart and cardiovascular system include the following:

- **Lipid profile or lipid panel:** This test is an analysis of cholesterol, HDL and LDL cholesterol, and triglycerides. Because research has shown that the most harmful type of LDL cholesterol is formed of small dense particles as opposed to larger, "fluffier" LDL particles, some physicians advise doing this more extensive test, while other physicians contend that the combination of low HDL-C, high LDL-C, and high triglycerides adequately predicts the presence of small, dense LDL-C particles. Discuss the need of this more advanced test with your doctor.

- **Complete blood count (CBC):** This test provides an analysis of various components of the blood, such as red and white blood cells. The CBC is used to diagnose anemia and to point to the need for other tests.

- **Glucose level:** This test serves as an analysis of insulin resistance and the possible presence of diabetes mellitus. Because insulin resistance and diabetes are risk factors for coronary heart disease (CHD), your physician closely monitors this result.

- **A basic or comprehensive metabolic panel:** This test provides an analysis of various factors related to kidney function, liver function, and electrolytes, which can be related to heart disease.

- **Thyroid level:** Your physician monitors this test for evidence of an overactive or underactive thyroid because such conditions can cause your heart to beat too rapidly or to increase the risk for CHD.

- **High sensitivity C-reactive protein (hs-CRP):** If you are at high risk of CHD or already have heart problems, your physician may wish to order this blood test, which detects inflammation in the blood vessels. Another inflammatory marker that your physician may choose to check is levels of fibrinogen.

Electrocardiogram (ECG)

Invented more than 100 years ago, the *electrocardiogram* (also called ECG or EKG) represents cardiology's first high-tech tool. But this graphic recording of the heart's electrical impulses remains one of the most useful tests. Many doctors include it as part of a routine annual physical exam to assess any potential heart problems. Most importantly, the ECG is an early diagnostic step taken when an individual exhibits symptoms that may indicate heart disease.

Currently, appropriate use criteria from a number of specialties such as the American College of Cardiology (ACC) and the American Heart Association (AHA) advise that ECGs are rarely appropriate for regular evaluation of healthy people without symptoms (those who rate low on global risk assessment scales). However, many physicians want at least a baseline ECG for a patient in case symptoms arise later. They also note that the percentage of American adults without at least one major risk factor for CHD is small. Used properly, ECGs can be useful tools; I suggest you discuss these issues and your circumstances fully with your doctor.

Exercise Stress Test

An exercise stress test, also called an *exercise tolerance test*, is an electrocardiogram that's administered while the heart is beating fast during exercise. After you're properly wired up, you're asked to walk and/or run at progressively higher speeds on a motorized treadmill or to pedal against steadily increasing resistance on a stationary cycle. These exercise activities cause the heart to speed up.

Among the most important clinical information that this test reveals is whether adequate blood flow is reaching the heart during exercise. Thus, the exercise tolerance test is extremely useful for people who have chest pain or other cardiac symptoms in making the diagnosis of coronary heart disease (CHD), angina, and in some instances, unstable angina. It may also be used for people with risk factors such as obesity, diabetes, or high blood pressure before beginning an exercise program. Appropriate use criteria suggest it is rarely appropriate for low-risk individuals who have no symptoms.

Echocardiogram

An *echocardiogram,* which also goes by the names *cardiac sonogram* and *cardiac ultrasound,* is a noninvasive test. It bounces sound waves off various structures of the heart. Sound waves are sent out by and then return to a device known as a transducer, which then converts them into a moving picture of all the structures of the heart.

Echocardiography gives a good picture of how well the heart is pumping blood, the condition and functioning of the heart valves, and whether there is any heart enlargement or thickening of the muscle walls. Echocardiograms are very useful for evaluating problems related to heart failure and atrial fibrillation as well as valve functioning. However, guidelines indicate that this test is rarely appropriate for healthy individuals who have no symptoms and have a low risk of CHD as measured by a valid global risk assessment tool.

Coronary Calcium Scan

Calcium in the arteries of the heart is an indication of *atherosclerosis*, the plaques that narrow the coronary arteries causing CHD. Finding calcium in the coronary arteries is useful in the early diagnosis of heart disease in individuals who are at moderate risk of heart disease, regardless of whether they have symptoms or not. Typically, moderate risk means having a 10 percent to 20 percent change of having a heart attack in the next ten years, based on a validated assessment tool. ACC and AHA guidelines do not recommend this test for routine screening for heart disease in individuals who have no symptoms and are at low risk.

The coronary calcium scan, also called *coronary calcium scoring*, uses computed tomography (often called a CT scan or CAT scan). CT scanning uses high-speed X-rays to create very precise images of the heart and large vessels leading to the heart. Because CT scans use radiation, pregnant women shouldn't have them. Whatever your status, be sure to discuss potential benefits, risks, and costs with your doctor.

Cardiac MRI

Cardiac magnetic resonance imaging (MRI) uses large magnets to create a powerful magnetic field that produces three-dimensional images (still and moving) of the heart and its structures. In recent years, research has increased the ways to use MRIs to help diagnose coronary heart disease as well as to indicate the condition of the heart muscle and the damage from a heart attack. However, because of the intense magnetic field, if you have a medical device such as an implanted defibrillator or pacemaker, MRIs are usually not for you. Since the uses of cardiac MRI are varied, make sure you discuss fully with your healthcare team what they are seeking to evaluate in your case.

Angiography

When a contrast material (often called a *dye*) is injected through a catheter to make arteries or other structures of the heart visible to X-rays, the procedure is called *angiography*. An advanced procedure, it usually is performed in a heart catheterization laboratory by a cardiologist who specializes in the field.

Patients undergo heart catheterizations to provide definitive evidence of any abnormalities that may be present

As a diagnostic test, heart catheterization is typically used when another less invasive cardiac test has indicated the probability of serious problems such as blocked coronary arteries. It is often used for this purpose in the presence of unstable angina or a heart attack to identify blockages. For example, most patients who undergo coronary artery bypass grafting and all patients who undergo angioplasty undergo heart catheterization first. Heart catheterization is a very serious procedure, and your doctor will discuss the reasons, benefits, and risks of it carefully with you.

Carotid Artery Ultrasound

The carotid arteries run up either side of your neck and carry oxygenated blood to the front of the brain. Atherosclerotic plaque narrowing these arteries is a risk factor for stroke.

Many direct-to-consumer "preventive screening" companies advertise these scans as a way to "put your mind at rest" or, should the ultrasound indicate narrowings, save you from a stroke. Unfortunately, to date there is inadequate evidence that such screenings in individuals without symptoms actually reduce strokes or save lives. In fact, such screenings produce a number of false positives. If you are worried that you may be at risk of a stroke or if you have had any symptoms of stroke, such as transient ischemic attacks (TIAs), consult your physician at once to discuss the right diagnostic approach for you. At present, no authoritative medical organization recommends this type of direct screenings.

Abdominal Aortic Aneurysm Ultrasound

An aneurysm is a bulge in the wall of a blood vessel. An aortic aneurysm occurs in the aorta, the large vessel that carries oxygenated blood from the heart to the rest of the body. Ruptured abdominal aortic aneurysms (AAA) are the primary cause of death in between 10,000 and 11,000 deaths a year in the U.S.

AAAs are most likely to occur in older white men who have ever smoked. Family history of AAA may also up the risk. For this reason, preventive guidelines recommend that men between 65 and 75 who are current or former smokers receive one ultrasound screening. Many direct-to-consumer screening companies also actively advertise this screening test to the general public. The guidelines, however, also recommend that the screening take place in an accredited facility with technologists who have appropriate credentials. If you think you may be at risk of AAA, discuss screening with your doctor.

Checking Out Other Cardiac Tests

The cardiac tests in this chapter just touch on the many tests that exist for cardiac and other health issues. You can find out more about cardiac tests at several reliable websites, including the following:

- ✔ MedlinePlus (www.medlineplus.gov), created by the U.S. National Library of medicine
- ✔ www.heart.org, the website of the American Heart Association
- ✔ www.cardiosource.org from the American College of Cardiology

Chapter 23

Ten Tips for Involving Your Family in a Heart-Healthy Lifestyle

*P*ursuing good health and preventing heart disease is most successful when it's a family affair. Whether you are just starting your family, in the midst of raising your children, exploring the newfound freedoms of empty nesters, or enjoying an extended family as grandparents, these ten pointers provide useful ideas you can adapt to your needs and situation.

Start Early

Health habits start in childhood. Active children usually become active adults. Children who learn to like a variety of nutritious foods and develop heart-healthy eating patterns typically follow those patterns as they grow into adults. Here are some suggestions:

✔ Start introducing a variety of vegetables and fruits to children when they start eating solid foods. When they graduate from strained or pureed foods, continue to introduce a variety of healthful foods.

You may need to offer a new food more than five or ten times before a child accepts it. Also, remember to use positive reinforcement, but don't use food as either a reward or a punishment.

✔ Play actively with young children indoors and out. As they grow older introduce fun activities that they can participate in: Take a walk after dinner or a short hike in the park. Tag, hide-and-seek, and red rover are enjoyable backyard games for everyone. As children grow and show interest in specific sports or activities, do what you can to enable their participation.

Model Healthful Behaviors

Children are natural copycats. Children who see parents (and older siblings) eating nutritious foods and being active are likely to copy those behaviors. Parents and older siblings can make a point to include younger members in outdoor activities and games and to take time to play with younger children doing the things they like best. Grandparents can also use these strategies. The heart-healthy approach to choosing foods and planning meals presented in Chapter 5 is appropriate for all members of the family who eat solid foods. Seeing parents and older siblings enjoy eating a variety of foods encourages younger children to try the same foods.

When you are tempted to bicycle without your helmet or down a big bag of chips while watching your favorite TV show, just remember young eyes are watching and learning.

Eat Together

Public "wisdom" may suggest that busy families are eating together less today than in the past. Happily, that trend has been reversed. More families today are eating at least four or five dinners together weekly than they were 15 years ago. That's a good thing. Children and adults who eat family dinners together tend to have better nutrient intakes and to eat more fruits and vegetables and other nutritious foods. Family members, particularly youth, tend to have better weight control.

Family dinners offer other benefits: They provide time for the family to share together. Teens report that catching up on what other members of the family are doing is the best part of these meals. Younger children are likely to feel more a part of the family and more secure. Children and youth who eat more meals together with their parents also tend to do better in school and have fewer behavioral problems, such as substance abuse.

Play Together

Getting adequate physical activity and exercise throughout the lifespan is one of the two most important things anyone can do for heart health and life-long well-being. The earlier you start, the better. Active children tend to grow into active adults. Regular exercise helps everyone maintain a healthy weight and build strong muscles and bones. Activity helps control cholesterol, blood pressure, and insulin resistance (prediabetes) — all risk factors for heart disease. In short, being physically active in childhood and thereafter, as the saying goes, adds years to your life and life to your years.

The family circle offers the best place to start establishing active habits. Children enjoy playing with parents and older siblings and relatives. They can hardly wait to begin doing things the "grownups" are doing. Can you remember, for example, how much you wanted your first bicycle? Planning activities that the whole family can participate in — from backyard games to hiking or biking trips — also helps children develop social skills, including how to work as a team, how to make decisions, and how to give leadership.

Limit Screen Time

Recommended TV viewing time for children over age 2 and up through adulthood is just one to two hours daily. Yet, on average, children in the United States watch three hours of TV daily. When other screen time, such as playing video games, surfing the Internet, or doing homework on the computer, is added in, average screen time rises to five to seven hours a day! Too much screen time is associated with a greater risk of overweight and obesity, irregular or inadequate sleep, and increased risk, in children, of attention problems, anxiety, and depression. More screen time typically means less physical activity.

Here are some strategies you can use to improve the situation (adults should set an example by also following these strategies):

- Cut off the TV except when you are watching shows planned in advance — no using TV for background sound.
- Keep TVs and computers out of bedrooms.
- Don't eat or snack while watching TV, playing video games, or using the computer (that goes for tablets and smartphones, too).

Involve Children in Making Meals and Planning Activities

It's never too early to start learning to make healthy choices and to begin developing the skills you need to carry out those choices. When it comes to trying new foods or dishes, for example, younger children are more likely to be receptive to trying foods that they have helped pick out in the grocery or to eat a food that they have helped make. We all think of the fun children have making cookies, for instance, but they can have as much fun making whole grain bread or pizza dough and preparing vegetables for cooking or putting in a salad.

Children are active by nature. Just think about the difficulty a 2-year-old (who is not sleepy) has sitting still. Structurally, the human body is designed to be in motion much of the time. Staying in motion is not a problem, either, when you are doing something you enjoy. So start early by engaging children in deciding what activities the family should do. Pay attention to which activities they enjoy most and provide opportunities for them to build on those activities. These strategies can reinforce the activity habit.

Get Plenty of Sleep

Sleep promotes a healthy immune system. Getting adequate sleep can also improve mood and cognitive function, including memory and learning. Just as important, adequate sleep helps your body function physically. Conversely, sleep deprivation can lower your ability to perform physical tasks safely, and it has been associated in a number of studies with a higher risk of developing health problems, such as heart disease, diabetes, and obesity.

How much sleep do you need? Needs vary from individual to individual, but almost everyone has a basic (or "basal") sleep need that falls within an average range. Following are some average daily sleep needs:

Recommended Hours of Sleep Daily	Age
16–18 hours	Newborns
11–12 hours	Preschoolers
At least 10 hours	School age children
9–10 hours	Teens
7–8 hours	Adults of all ages, including older adults

Support Each Other

Medical science clearly shows that having adequate social support from family and friends helps people who have had a heart attack recover and helps people who have coronary heart disease manage their health more positively. Research also suggests, however, that having low social support increases the risk of developing heart disease by 1.5 to 2 times, even for healthy individuals.

In my own medical practice, I have observed the importance to general health and management of heart conditions of having both a circle of support and meaningful ways to be of support to others. Social support is a two-way street — you give and you receive. What better place to explore the benefits of sharing positively and supportively than within the family?

Many people also have an important "third place" (beyond family and work) that provides meaning and a community of support in their lives. Such places include faith communities, volunteer groups that benefit the community, sports, garden, hobby, or social clubs or groups, and many more.

Start Where You Are Today

Okay, what if it's too late to start early with your kids — they're teens not toddlers? Or what if you are empty nesters? It may sound simplistic, but you start where you — and your family — are. Take one step at a time and add additional steps as you can. Here are just a few suggestions of the variety of steps you can begin to take to encourage heart-healthy living wherever your family currently is:

- If you eat only two dinners a week together as a family, add one more family meal.
- Add one more vegetable to dinner.
- Take a heart-healthy lunch two days a week rather than eating out every day.
- Take fruit or nuts rather than chips or a candy bar for a snack.
- Take a walk as a family one evening after dinner or on a weekend day.
- Sit down with the whole family and add goals for more activity. Plan an active weekend trip or vacation. Increase these types of steps as you can.

If just you and your spouse or partner are at home, start to listen more actively today to how you can be more supportive. Maybe it's time to sit down and discuss what you two can do together to help one another and how you can get more enjoyment out of your time together as you practice heart-healthy living.

Never Confuse "Lapse" with "Collapse"

At some point, as you pursue a good health goal, you'll take an awkward step or fall back into an old practice. Maybe one week when your spouse is on a business trip and every child has an evening school activity, the family doesn't manage even one dinner or evening walk together, and it seems like there's no opportunity or time to fix nutritious lunches to take to work or school. To top the problem off, the next week seems just as challenging. The temptation is to give up the effort.

In many years of medical practice working with patients on making heart-healthy lifestyle changes, I have seen more people fail because they treated a lapse of a week or two as a total collapse and gave up. A lapse, however, is temporary. Working for heart health is a cumulative activity for you and each member of the family. So it's important not to place blame, to accept the occasional lapse, and to just get going again, picking up where you left off.

I'll also share a final secret: The single most important reason that individuals and families lapse and collapse is that they try to make too many changes at once. If that happens to you and your family, pause and rethink your goals and make sure that you are building slowly. It takes time to make healthy practices a daily habit.

Appendix

Metric Conversion Guide

● ●

*N**ote:* The recipes in this book weren't developed or tested using metric measurements. There may be some variation in quality when converting to metric units.

Common Abbreviations

Abbreviation(s)	What It Stands For
cm	Centimeter
C., c.	Cup
G, g	Gram
kg	Kilogram
L, l	Liter
lb.	Pound
mL, ml	Milliliter
oz.	Ounce
pt.	Pint
t., tsp.	Teaspoon
T., Tb., Tbsp.	Tablespoon

Volume

U.S. Units	Canadian Metric	Australian Metric
¼ teaspoon	1 milliliter	1 milliliter
½ teaspoon	2 milliliters	2 milliliters
1 teaspoon	5 milliliters	5 milliliters
1 tablespoon	15 milliliters	20 milliliters

(continued)

Volume *(continued)*

U.S. Units	Canadian Metric	Australian Metric
¼ cup	50 milliliters	60 milliliters
⅓ cup	75 milliliters	80 milliliters
½ cup	125 milliliters	125 milliliters
⅔ cup	150 milliliters	170 milliliters
¾ cup	175 milliliters	190 milliliters
1 cup	250 milliliters	250 milliliters
1 quart	1 liter	1 liter
1½ quarts	1.5 liters	1.5 liters
2 quarts	2 liters	2 liters
2½ quarts	2.5 liters	2.5 liters
3 quarts	3 liters	3 liters
4 quarts (1 gallon)	4 liters	4 liters

Weight

U.S. Units	Canadian Metric	Australian Metric
1 ounce	30 grams	30 grams
2 ounces	55 grams	60 grams
3 ounces	85 grams	90 grams
4 ounces (¼ pound)	115 grams	125 grams
8 ounces (½ pound)	225 grams	225 grams
16 ounces (1 pound)	455 grams	500 grams (½ kilogram)

Length

Inches	Centimeters
0.5	1.5
1	2.5
2	5.0
3	7.5
4	10.0
5	12.5

Inches	Centimeters
6	15.0
7	17.5
8	20.5
9	23.0
10	25.5
11	28.0
12	30.5

Temperature (Degrees)	
Fahrenheit	Celsius
32	0
212	100
250	120
275	140
300	150
325	160
350	180
375	190
400	200
425	220
450	230
475	240
500	260

Index

About the Author

Dr. Rippe is a graduate of Harvard College and Harvard Medical School with postgraduate training at Massachusetts General Hospital. He is the founder and director of Rippe Lifestyle Institute and Professor of Biomedical Science at the University of Central Florida. Dr. Rippe is also founder and director of Rippe Health Evaluation in Orlando, Florida.

Dr. Rippe is regarded as one of the leading authorities on preventive cardiology, health and fitness, and healthy weight loss in the United States. Under his leadership, the Rippe Lifestyle Institute has conducted numerous research projects on cardiovascular risk-factor reduction, fitness walking, weight loss, sports training, cholesterol reduction, and low-fat diets. Laboratory members have presented more than 275 papers at national, medical, and scientific meetings in the last 25 years. Dr. Rippe has written more than 400 publications on issues in medicine, health and fitness, and weight management. He has also written or edited 49 books, including 31 medical texts and 18 books on health and fitness for the general public. *Fitness Walking* (Perigee, 1985) and *Fitness Walking for Women* (Perigee, 1987) were recipients of National American Health Book Awards. More recent books include The *Healthy Heart For Dummies* (Wiley, 1999), *The Healthy Heart Cookbook For Dummies* (Wiley, 2000, 2011), *Heart Disease For Dummies* (Wiley, 2004), *Your Plan for a Balanced Life* (Thomas Nelson, 2007), *High Performance Health* (Thomas Nelson, 2007) and *High Performance Health Workbook* (Thomas Nelson, 2007). For more on Dr. Rippe's publications see `http://www.rippelifestyle.com`.

Dr. Rippe also edits a major academic textbook, *Lifestyle Medicine* (2nd Ed., CRC Press, 2013), the first textbook to guide physicians in the diverse aspects of how to incorporate lifestyle recommendations into the practice of modern medicine. His intensive-care textbook, *Irwin and Rippe's Intensive Care Medicine* (7th edition, 2011; co-edited with Dr. Richard Irwin), is the world's leading textbook on intensive and coronary care. Dr. Rippe edits the *American Journal of Lifestyle Medicine,* the only peer-reviewed medical journal in lifestyle medicine (SAGE, 2007–present). He is also Editor-in-Chief of a two-volume *Encyclopedia of Lifestyle Medicine and Health* (SAGE, 2012).

Dr. Rippe's work has been featured on *The Today Show*, *Good Morning America*, PBS's *Bodywatch,* CBS Morning and Evening News, and CNN, and in a variety of print media, including *The New York Times, New York Times Magazine, L.A. Times, The Wall Street Journal*, and many monthly publications. He comments regularly on health and fitness for *USA Today, American Health,* and *Prevention.* He served for three years as Medical Editor for the Television Food Network (TVFN).

A lifelong and avid athlete, Dr. Rippe maintains his personal fitness with a regular swim, walk, jog, and weight-training program. He holds a black belt in karate and is an avid windsurfer, skier, and tennis player. He lives outside of Boston with his wife, television news anchor Stephanie Hart, and their four children, Hart, Jaelin, Devon, and Jamie.

Dedication

To Stephanie, Hart, Jaelin, Devon, and Jamie, who make my heart sing and provide the cornerstone for my personal program to maintain a healthy heart.

Author's Acknowledgments

It would be impossible to cite all of the individuals who have provided advice and support during the time it took to complete this book. However, several deserve special recognition for their significant contributions.

First, I would like to acknowledge and applaud the superb writing and editorial skills of my main collaborator, Mary Abbott Waite. As we updated and refocused this new edition as *Preventing & Reversing Heart Disease For Dummies* (the successor to *Heart Disease For Dummies*, 2004) Mary Abbott has taken complex medical topics and edited my thoughts in a way that makes the message clear, concise, and user-friendly.

Second, my Editorial Director Beth Grady and Executive Assistant Carol Moreau provided splendid support to me and to Mary Abbott to help us keep this whole process moving forward in the midst of busy schedules.

I also would like to commend and thank top chefs from across America who wrote the recipes that are included in this book from *The Healthy Heart Cookbook For Dummies*. These include Paul Agnelli, Hans Bergmann, MaryAnn Saporito Boothroyd, Ignatius Chang, Garrett Cho, Alfonso Constriciani, Dale R. Gussett, Kevin T. Jones, Constantin Kerageorgiou, Joe Mannke, Melanie Mulcahy, Amy Myrdal, Carrie Nahabedian, Bradley Ogden, Alvaro Ojeda and Laura Maioglio, Marcus Samuelson, Kimberly Shaker, RoxSand Suarez, Mark Tarbell, and Chris Toole and Sandra Holland. Thanks also go to authors Meri Raffetto, RD, and Wendy Jo Peterson, MS RD, who created the recipes which appear in this book from the *Mediterranean Diet Cookbook*.

I am also indebted to the talented research staff at my laboratory, the Rippe Lifestyle Institute in Shrewsbury, Massachusetts, and Celebration, Florida. Under the superb direction of Research Director Ted Angelopoulos, PhD, MPH, our staff of health-care and research professionals have all provided useful insights and ongoing clinical validation of many of the concepts discussed in this book.

My professional colleagues have been a source of continuing intellectual stimulation throughout my career as a cardiologist. I would like to particularly acknowledge Dr. Joseph Alpert, Chief of Medicine at the University of Arizona; Dr. Ira Ockene, Professor of Medicine and Director of the Preventive Cardiology program at UMass Medical School; and Dr. Richard S. Irwin, Professor of Medicine and Chair, Critical Care Operations, UMass Medical School and Memorial Medical Center.

Last, but certainly not least, my darling wife, Stephanie Hart Rippe, has provided the safe harbor without which none of these voyages, literary or otherwise, would be conceivable. While supporting my intense work schedule and often outlandish travel arrangements, she has grounded me with her love and inspired me with her courage, beauty, and intelligence. In addition, she has given me four beautiful daughters: Hart Elizabeth Rippe, Jaelin Davis Rippe, Devon Marshall Rippe, and Jamie Conrad Rippe. These five individuals who together comprise the "Rippe Women" continue to make it all worthwhile and have convinced me that I'm not only the luckiest but also the most-loved man in the universe.

To all of these individuals and many others who have helped along the way, my heartfelt gratitude. I hope the final product reflects the strength, commitment, and caring of all those who made it possible. In a small way, I hope that this book helps people who are either engaged in an ongoing battle against the number one killer in our country — heart disease — or who are seeking to prevent it, by providing useful facts, information, and above all motivation to live a heart-healthy lifestyle.

Publisher's Acknowledgments

Senior Acquisitions Editor: Tracy Boggier

Project Editor: Tracy L. Barr

Technical Editor: Joseph Alpert, MD

Art Coordinator: Alicia B. South

Project Coordinator: Melissa Cossell

Illustrator: Kathryn Born

Cover Image: © iStock.com/Inkout